D1234632

THE ROSETTA STONE OF THE HUMAN MIND

BF
38
S225
2007
Van

THE ROSETTA STONE OF THE HUMAN MIND

Three languages to integrate neurobiology and psychology

Vincenzo R. Sanguineti M.D.

Associate Professor, Psychiatry
Jefferson Medical College
Philadelphia

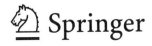 Springer

Cover insert: "Secret Translations in the Brain: from the magic of the neurons to the magic of creativity, as Art, Music, and Science; and the multilingual key to decode the mystery" by artist Nenne Sanguineti Poggi.

Library of Congress Control Number: 2006923487

ISBN-10: 0-387-33644-3   e-ISBN-10: 0-387-33645-1
ISBN-13: 978-0-387-33644-2

Printed on acid-free paper.

© 2007 Springer Science+Business Media, LLC
All rights reserved. This work may not be translated or copied in whole or in part without the written permission of the publisher (Springer Science+Business Media, LLC, 233 Spring Street, New York, NY 10013, USA), except for brief excerpts in connection with reviews or scholarly analysis. Use in connection with any form of information storage and retrieval, electronic adaptation, computer software, or by similar or dissimilar methodology now known or hereafter developed is forbidden.
The use in this publication of trade names, trademarks, service marks and similar terms, even if they are not identified as such, is not to be taken as an expression of opinion as to whether or not they are subject to proprietary rights.

Printed in the United States of America.

9 8 7 6 5 4 3 2 1

springer.com

For questioning is the piety of thought
(M. Heidegger, 1977, p. 35)

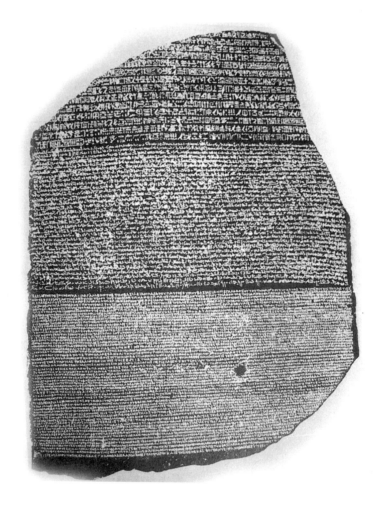

The Rosetta Stone in the British Museum
(Eastern Egyptian Gallery)
© The British Museum

Contents

Foreword

I met Vincenzo Sanguineti at a crucial point of my career, when, after 20 years of involvement in biological research applied to psychiatric disorders, I started to feel the emptiness and aridity of biological explanations that, besides the evidence of being incomplete and rough, lack, as Mandell stated, "the beauty and generativity of premolecular research." I realized that microscopic dissection had been the main objective of too many scientists, including myself, for too long and this attitude precluded us from developing a vision of the brain and of the mind in their entirety. Obviously, I do not reject neuroscience, I am still a neuroscientist, but now I know that neuroscience can provide me only with methods and not explanations. Meeting Vincenzo Sanguineti was an event that shaped my next steps, a bifurcation point, and the ensuing results were very fruitful, in that we arranged together two courses at the national meetings of the American Psychiatric Association that were a great success. On those occasions I could appreciate his broad mind and deep knowledge of neuroanatomy, neurophysiology, and neurochemistry, and his expressed discomfort with the current existence of only a few theories of the mind and the fact that psychoanalysts and neuroscientists are often too dogmatic and closed in their own convictions to be able to cooperate in a positive way.

Therefore, I was not surprised when I received his new book, *The Rosetta Stone to the Human Mind: Three Languages to Integrate Psychology and Neurobiology*, because I knew that he cultivates the intent to explain the complexity of the mind from different perspectives that are not mutually exclusive. He shows that they simply represent the use of different languages to describe the same entity.

Obviously, this book is only an attempt to do so, and Vincenzo Sanguineti is very modest and underlines this aspect, but with no doubt it is a serious and exhaustive attempt toward the holistic comprehension of that complexity that is the human mind. For this reason, probably, he forced himself to be simple, but not simplistic, so that the book might be understood by both neuroscientists and psychiatrists, coming as they do from different backgrounds. In addition, it is full of historical and literary references, as well as being in part centered on the myth of Eros and Psyche, with fascinating results.

Donatella Marazziti
Professor, Department of Psychiatry, Neurobiology,
        Pharmacology and Biotechnology, University of Pisa.
Director, Laboratory of Psychopharmacology, University of Pisa.
Author of *La Natura dell' Amore* (*The Nature of Love*, 2002).

Foreword

Over the past decade or so it has been my pleasure to help with the organization of and take part in several academic conferences and workshops in the general area of consciousness studies. Although I write pleasure, because there were opportunities to take in unfamiliar ideas and form new friendships, these experiences shared a frustrating feature that stemmed from the limited perspectives of the attendees.

For all our vaunted devotion to learning, we academics are a narrow lot with two major character flaws. First, we tend to favor the perspectives of reductionism. Overly impressed with the successes of the natural sciences, biologists, psychologists, psychiatrists, sociologists, economists, cultural anthropologists, and even philosophers mold their disciplines with the same bottom-up logical character that works so well in physics and even some simpler branches of chemistry. This tendency persists in the face of what seems overwhelming evidence to the contrary from the humanities, not to mention the events of a normal day or a normal life. Second, academics don't listen. Each one goes to a conference with the aim of convincing others that his point of view should prevail. Thus an interdisciplinary conference often collapses into a group of people talking past each other, generating impressive wind but little more. Of course I exaggerate here; many academics do listen to other perspectives and sincerely criticize their own, but not enough for the sounds of that wind to quiet.

And listen we must. Opening the doors to an appreciation of human spirit is now—as for many centuries—a central endeavor of our species, and it is becoming clear that no single perspective has a full set of keys. As people from different subcultures speak in diverse tongues, the first task that we face is to learn how to translate from one set of assumptions and jargon to those of another group. It is to this task that The *Rosetta Stone to the Human Mind* is directed.

   Working at a level that transcends individual academic disciplines, Dr. Sanguineti sees three main subcultures that need to be introduced to each other. The first of these is mathematical science, with its ancient traditions, curious logic, and symbolic jottings that seem meaningless except to those who (strangely) find them exciting. Second is the subjective domain, from where we retrieve descriptions of that inner space that we call our psyche and that finds its finest expression in the arts, which predate recorded human history and continue to fascinate and confuse (not necessarily in that order) those trained in the sciences. Yet art springs directly from spirit and cries to be heard. Finally, there are observations of human mind and spirit by those who deal directly with it without preconceived limits on what they are allowed to see: the author's "objective observers."

   The languages of these three—the theorist, the artist, and the objective observer—are interpreted in terms of each other by Dr. Sanguineti in this thoughtful book and used to create a metalanguage with sufficient depth to comprehend the nature of the human mind. It is a remarkable achievement, which all who wonder will profit from reading and cherish.

Alwyn Scott
Emeritus Professor, Department of Mathematics, University of Arizona.
Professor, Department of Informatics and Mathematical
   Modeling, Technical University of Denmark.
Author of *Stairway to the Mind: The Controversial New
   Science of Consciousness* (1995); *Nonlinear Science:
   Emergence and Dynamics of Coherent Structures* (1999);
   Neuroscience: A Mathematical Primer* (2002).

Foreword

How do the following words relate to one another: mind, soul, self, spirit, identity, character, subject, person, personality, psyche, individual, ego, consciousness, brain, I? In no other field of human investigation does such a rich proliferation of mysteries unfold from beneath the simplest question. Scientists who investigate the brain may be perfectly happy to admit that their methods are very different from those of psychoanalysts, priests, philosophers, and poets, but is it as easy to be certain that each of these thinkers is actually investigating the same thing? Is the brain consciousness? Is consciousness the subject? Is the ego the self? An irreducible complexity emerges not only between the languages used to explain human interior life, but even between their differing ways of conceiving of their object. Even when there is a clear sense of the differences between these various terms, the relationship between them remains mysterious. How does the spirit connect with the brain, for example? And where exactly is "the self"?

Yet it is no easy matter to solve this disproportion by establishing an objective hierarchy of the more or less objective, the more or less hypothetical, or the more or less abstract. There is no ultimate theory of the self that will overrule or supplant all the others, and each one that aspires to this title soon reveals its limitations and provokes even more, often unanswerable questions. None of our many discourses of subjectivity can be ruled out absolutely as totally inappropriate or useless. Chemical therapy may prove profitable for a wide range of psychological conditions, but useless for the obscure abstract spiritual crisis; philosophers may puzzle over a weakening self-concept that behavioral modification therapy can allow to be managed. Science may aspire in the objective modeling of brain-function, at the expense of the representation of contingent lived experience. And all of this leaves aside the question of whether interior life is indeed a "problem" that can be met by a solution, an object that can be modeled, or a question that can be answered.

In the present book, Vincenzo Sanguineti accepts the many challenges of this situation head on, by refusing to settle for a simple, single approach as the ultimate methodology. The key themes of his study revolve around complexity, inclusiveness, and metaphoricity. First, interior life is so irreducibly complex and unstable that no final explanation or model of it will be possible. This not only resonates with the exploratory nature of thought, and the fact that so little consensus has been reached, but also with the open-endedness and wide-ranging possibilities of the subjectivity of daily life. Second, no single theory will ever achieve the status of the key to all (subjective) mythologies. The integration of different approaches—or at least the open conversation between them—beckons as the necessary path that will allow, not only for workable solutions to individuals who have to deal with biochemical imbalances but also uncertainties about culturally constituted identities and immediate human relationships. Finally, as he says (p. 87): "Choose your preferred metaphor"! The process of modeling can never reduce to zero its dependence on abstract, even fictional imagery and language as a way of allowing its insights to be represented. Whether it takes the form of diagrams, graphs, models, images, illustrations or labels, metaphor always plays a function in the revelation of the self. This practice finds its most happy example in the choice of the Rosetta Stone itself as the metaphor for the way different languages cohabit the same investigative space of the quest for understanding who or what we are.

Yet, even this usage leads to even more questions. The history of the reception of the Rosetta Stone required that the three languages be read for what they had in common. They were clues to each other, allowing obscure symbols to reveal their unknown significance. Yet, anyone who has experienced the liminal space where one language meets another is aware of the untranslatable dimension that divides one symbolic order from another. The three languages on the Rosetta Stone cannot be reduced to a single meaning, because this meaning will be at the cost of the minute but inescapable differences in tone, emphasis, and timbre that separate individual languages. What is it in each of these languages that cannot be translated into the others? The achievement of this book is to capture the complexity of the integration of different conceptual languages: What do they say together but what does each of them say that cannot be translated into the others? Where do they overlap, and where do they need the unique idiosyncratic contribution that only each particular language can provide?

What this ambitious project captures is the necessary, inalienable mystery of the self, the fact that each of our languages for it remains provisional and open. Yet far from being locked in the domain of the religious, the obscure and the esoteric, this mystery is connected with the rigours of scientific investigation and intellectual analysis. To me, this seems appropriate to the task: only the full, unreserved powers of the human intellect in all its variety can deal with the mystery of the human self, without ever absolutely reducing the awe, curiosity and sense of open-ended challenge it will always provoke.

Nick Mansfield
Associate Professor in Critical and Cultural Studies
    Division of Society, Culture, Media and Philosophy
    Macquarie University.
Author of *Subjectivity: Theories of the Self from Freud to*
    Haraway (2000); *Cultural Studies and Critical Theory*
    (with Patrick Fuery, 2000); *Masochism: The Art of Power*
    (1997); *Cultural Studies and the New Humanities:*
    Concepts and Controversies (with Patrick Fuery, 1997);
    To Die of Desire (1993).

Foreword

The subject of consciousness has been and still is an enigma to the inquiring minds of multiple disciplines over the centuries. It has been addressed by poetry, art, and song; by myth, legend, theology, philosophy, and rational systems of classification; by psychology and psychoanalysis; and, more recently, by theoretical physics and the mathematics of quantum mechanics and nonlinear dynamics.

As has been stated by Dr. Sanguineti, the "bottom up" approach, although erudite, not only falls short but frankly is devoid of that *elan vital* that signifies the successful illumination of a complex question. Therefore, there has been no "Eureka! We have found it!" epiphany that signifies or marks that the essence and core of an issue has at last been discovered. All of the above has led science to grudgingly deal with the much resisted enigma of subjectivity itself. This step requires a paradigm jump from intellect to spirit, from content to context, and away from the myopic literalness of the Newtonian system that condemns knowledge to the constraints of the epistemological blindness consequent to the limitation of the principles of causality and form.

Subjectivity is of a different domain. It is that of nonlinear context rather than linear content and the realm of noncausal reality. Newtonian description is always "about" and external to that which is described and is therefore devoid of essence or experience. We "talk about" the so-called objective, but we live completely, totally, and wholly within the ubiquitous, nonstop, alwaysness, and continuous nowness of the all-embracing subjectivity of existence itself.

The investigation of the immense "phase-space" of the human psyche has largely been like exploration without a compass, much less a global positioning system. In fact, researchers have not even been aware of what level of consciousness they were talking about nor was there a way to verify either discoveries or the suitability of even the investigative tools that were being hopefully relied upon (e.g., mathematics, intellect, reason, semantics, etc.). Dr. Sanguineti gets to the crux of the problem by stating that "humans do not

xviii   *Foreword*

have any real sense of the profundity and intricacy of their minds, nor are
they taught to identify the streams of collective data and affective states that
participate to their own being" (p. 134). This is in agreement with our own
published research, which documents that the unenlightened human mind is
usually unable to discern truth from falsehood.

Actually, recent discoveries from this research about verifiable, quantifiable
levels of consciousness allow us to establish common reference points that
demystify and clarify the traditionally obscure realms of subjectivity. For
instance, on the 1:1000 Scale of the Levels of Consciousness that we use for
our research, truth "calibrates" at 200, the intellect is in the 400s, and the higher
human qualities of compassion, love, joy, peace, and excellence are in the
500s. Level 600 denotes the unusual but remarkable level traditionally termed
enlightenment. (The scale was based on the discovery of how to tell truth from
falsehood and delineate the realms of the false from the true, of power versus
force, of spiritual from intellectual, and of illuminated states of gnosis from
merely intellectual positionalities and presumptions.)

In essence, the research cited above addresses the pressing need to recon-
textualize the study of the human psyche. Critical to this reframing is the
demonstration of the relationship of content (linear), and context (nonlinear),
and the critical clarification that the truth of any statement can only be of
varying degrees which are powerfully determined by the usually unstated,
ignored, undefined, or naively presumed context.

As Dr. Sanguineti concludes from his courageous exploratory plunge into
the historic phantasmagoria of the human psyche, the recognition of the
sovereignty of subjectivity is the great missing link and, therefore, the crucial
reality that has eluded conventional scientific explanations of such a vast
and seemingly undecipherable challenge as the human psyche. The subjective
experience of reading Dr. Sanguineti's *Rosetta Stone* was quite interesting and
relatively unique. At the conclusion of reading most books, there is a feeling of
conclusion, a sort of "Well, that's that" finalization that the subject matter has
supplied information and now the experience of its perusal is over and relatively
"done with." This book resulted in an altogether different response in that, at
its conclusion, there was the feeling of having really just started to understand
its content. I found myself rereading the book, which, in itself, is quite
unusual. The material is presented in a freewheeling style instead of the usual
progressive constraint of some epistemological positionality or conventional
manner of subject presentation. This turned out to be quite productive. For
example, I just had to check out the validity of the cited ancient Egyptians'
realization that the "Ka" is the spirit body that is concordant with the physical
body and leaves it to continue on as life after physical death. This "Ka" is the
energy body of consciousness, and, as research confirmed, it is the locus of the
centralizing sense of "I-ness." Research indicates that subjective awareness,

out of which any capacity to "know" arises, is a faculty of the *etheric* brain, not the physical one (e.g., the Ka is noumenal, science is phenomenal). To progress, consciousness research therefore has to transcend the limitation of the intellect and affirm the internal core reality of the self and not just the perceptual delineation of the ego.

How do we know that statement to be true? Because the Ka of the reader already knows it by gnosis. Dr. Sanguineti's book inspires one to break the chains and slavery of neural chemistry and its horrible microtubules. Escape to freedom—the Ka is immortal and laughs at puny physicality and the egomania of the intellect.

The evolution of consciousness is conclusively and provably transcendent. When, through meditation and spiritual endeavor, the identification with the ego of the individual self ceases, then the radical subjectivity of the divinity of the "I" of the self shines forth and the illusion of a separate personal self dissolves into the ultimate context which is the very source of awareness and existence itself. The presence is overwhelming, total, and outside of time. The self replaces the illusory self and the mind goes permanently silent. The condition is total and, in most cases, the subject retires from the world. Accordingly, after many years, the capacity to speak of the condition may return. The *ineffable* is neither definable nor describable and is of a different domain. To be at one with allness leaves nothing to speak about; to truly "know" is to "be." One cannot *know* thy self but only *be* thy self.

David R. Hawkins, M.D., Ph.D.
Director, Institute for Advanced Spiritual Research, Sedona, AZ.
Author of *Orthomolecular Psychiatry* (with Linus Pauling, 1973);
    Power versus Force: The Hidden Determinants of Human Behavior
    (1998); *The Eye of the I: From Which Nothing Is Hidden* (2001);
    and *I, Reality and Subjectivity* (2003).

Introduction

In 1799, while working at the reconstruction of Fort St. Julien, north of the little town of Rashid on the left bank of what in ancient times had been called the Bolbitinic arm of the river Nile, a French soldier in the Napoleonic army dislodged a large slab of black basalt covered with carvings (Budge, 1989).

The stone was taken to Cairo and eventually examined by archaeologists and Egyptologists accompanying the French army at Bonaparte's expressed request. They quickly realized that the slab of basalt carried a "trilingual" message (actually, inscriptions in two languages and three alphabets). The first was in ideograms, the pictorial and as yet bewildering "hieroglyphs" that were still baffling all those who attempted to translate them. The second inscription was carved in "demotic" Egyptian, the colloquial writing system of ancient Egypt. The third inscription was written in ancient Greek. After reading the Greek passage it became clear that the stone carried an invaluable gift: the same text written in hieroglyphs, demotic Egyptian, and Greek.

The slab was to be shipped to France for display in the Louvre, but Napoleon was defeated by the British, and the stone was shipped to London instead. Named the Rosetta Stone from the place of its unearthing (Rosetta being the European name for Rashid), it is still on display in the British Museum, one of the most important archaeological discoveries of all time. Eventually, by integrating the information on the same phenomenon described in the three very diverse alphabets, the secrets imbedded in the Egyptian hieroglyphs gradually became apparent. The exquisite images became verbal sounds that reflect the everyday language of the Egyptian people, and the depth and complexity of that ancient culture was slowly revealed, making humanity that much richer in the process.

The pictorial alphabet had been the tool of expression of the religious-political system of ancient Egypt. Its invention was attributed to the God Thoth, "the heart and tongue" of the sun god Ra, and it carried instructions on how to deal with the universal themes of gods, death, and the afterlife. It recorded the deeds of the men-gods—the pharaohs—and of the main religious-political rulers of the country. It appeared to have nothing in common with the demotic writing of the people, characterized by a set of signs, each representing a specific sound or "letter." And yet the demotic character proved to be an abbreviated and modified form of the hieratic character, a cursive form of hieroglyphic writing. The pictures of humans and animals, objects and cryptic symbols were representations of the same basic sounds conveyed by their demotic counterparts.

It needs to be noted that even with a three-alphabet translation of the text obstacles to their use kept creeping up, now largely related to jealousy and competitiveness among experts, some of whom were apparently driven by the desire to be known as the repositories of the true translation, the discoverers of the key to the real alphabet.

In the present book I will introduce a different sort of Rosetta Stone: three languages (actually, it may be more correct even in our case to speak of two languages and three alphabets) which, when used conjointly, may significantly facilitate the understanding of psyche.

The first language is the language of physics and mathematics. It addresses the system of rules that potentially organize and direct the universality of bios, or life, that vast conglomerate of all biological organisms, of which humanity is just one specific form. The other two languages may actually be considered as different alphabets of a common domain, that of neuropsychobiology. These two languages address a specific phenomenon, the human brain and the human mind. The information is usually presented in two different forms: the objective, observer-related language of neurobiology (commonly identified with the field of neuroscience) and the first-person, subjective language of the individual mind (commonly identified with the field of psychology).

The scope of my writing is to illustrate the advantages that might be derived from using these three languages to understand diverse aspects of the mind. For each language I will employ a specific model, one with which I have become acquainted in the course of my search for a method to enable me to decipher the human subject. We are all preferentially versed in the language and symbols that are the common modes of expression for our specific fields of interest, for those areas in which we spend most of our professional lives. These predilections may induce either the idea that our language is the one best fitted to give accurate descriptions (while other languages appear imprecise or incomplete), or that others are not able to use it as accurately as we do; or, frequently, a combination of the above. I therefore need to repeat the statement that my focus is *the versatility aspect*, the advantage to be gained from providing ourselves and becoming acquainted with a Rosetta Stone of sorts. In the same vein, I do not want to suggest that the specific models I use are the final ones. On the contrary, I am of the opinion that we are still very tentative and limited in our attempts to understand mind. In this respect, we continue to be the blind men around the elephant.

The mathematical language model that I have chosen goes under the label of *nonlinear dynamics* and I will liberally use the information on this language provided by neuroscientist and mathematician Alwyn Scott (2002). To illustrate the demotic, first-person language, I have relied on the mythological model of Psyche as reported in substantial detail by lecturer and philosopher Apuleius. The observer-centered language models I have selected are those of neuroscientists Gerald Edelman (1989, 1992; Edelman & Tononi, 2000) and Antonio Damasio (1994, 1999), and also in this case I will liberally use the information provided by these experts.

In the first part of the book I will describe these languages in some detail as I understand them. I emphasize the understanding part in order to underscore the fact that all these languages are understandable by lay people. A good point to start from is to realize that they all mean the same thing; they are simply expressing different metaphors that emerge from the creative phase space (see Chapter 2) of specific human minds. Rather than being looked at with diffidence they should be approached with curiosity and with the expectation that they may yield invaluable information.

Part II presents selected mental phenomena, as they appear when translated into each language. By superimposing these translations the mental phenomena assume greater depth and definition: this is congruent with the fact that the phenomena are now observed from a three-dimensional rather than a one-dimensional perspective.

In the final section I will touch upon some examples of how this composite knowledge can enhance our understanding of the human mind, not only at the individual level but also in a broader sociocultural context. Finally, this book has to be taken for what it really is: an admittedly naive exercise in the integration of the different approaches used to probe the mystery of mind; and nothing more.

The Puzzle

I am on a dirt road twisting its way through hills of a light-brown color, with sparse dusty bushes and small trees. The road at times is larger, and then I drive my champagne spider Alfa Romeo with the top down. At times the road gets narrow, almost a trail, and then I put my Alfa in my left pocket and proceed on foot. She[1] does not seem to mind the shift in states, is willing to go along, and ready to carry me on when the road allows me to let her "do the going." I take my time looking at the birds and at the countryside. Most of the birds in flight are to my right; some perch on the small trees at both sides of the road. I know that in a roundabout way the road brings me *also* to Thebes; anyway it has to do with Thebes. This is definitely a Theban landscape.

A statement has been made, at the beginning of my journey: "You should find Oedipus before he reaches the crossing, and stop him from getting there." I am perfectly aware of the crossing to which the statement alludes, and the drama that is connected with it. At that crossing Laius' carriage will strike Oedipus, his unknown son. The son will then kill the father and go on to marry his own mother, thus fulfilling the nemesis cast on his ancestors by the gods. From that day on the drama will be reenacted in every son's psyche and come to represent—maybe—the inescapable pathway of human psychological development.[2]

My outlook is, though, fairly casual. As I go along, among the Boetian hills, my mental attitude is that if I meet Oedipus I *might* delay him, but I am not making myself hurry up, searching for him in order to reshape human destiny! Subliminally, I know that in an older dimension than the present one

---

[1] In Italian a car is feminine, and anyway I always relate to my Alfa as "she." Driving her is subtly sensuous and requires a sort of merging with her. It is an elegant, "slender," passionate, "petit" encounter in which she can always come up with some unpredictability; quite different from driving a Buick or an RV, where bigness and power are all that counts, all that is requested.

[2] Aggression around sexual dominance and sex as a reward. Keep this motif in mind.

the meeting and the slaying have already happened and yet I am also aware that I *could* seek a different outcome, should the situation offer itself.

As I reach the top of another hill through another trail—the Alfa in my pocket, the downhill side always on my left, as it has been for the entire journey, and birds still intermittently flying to my right![3]—I wake up.

My first "conscious" thought is that my recent enhanced proclivity and curiosity to consider other psychological developments than the Freudian one must have continued to operate in my brain during sleep, with a quite significant metaphorical outcome. I am also immediately aware that the dream is concurrently—and primarily—a piece of personal analysis superimposed on evolutionary blueprints.

As a rapidly expanding universe, the major dimensions of my life encapsulated in the dream unfold one after the other—or better, simultaneously: the Greek mythical heroes and the hubris/nemesis theme, the African landscapes (inclusive of birds!) closely reproduced in the "Theban" ones, the theme of the father, the reliance on intuition, my relationship to the feminine side (my adaptable Alfa) are just a few amongst the many (for a more detailed description of these specific dimensions see Sanguineti, 1999). Although decades ago my position concerning dreams—when I knew practically nothing about them—was quite skeptical, I now have so much exposure to them from countless encounters in the clinical arena that all doubts about their representing very meaningful expressions of the self (independent of any major ego interference) have completely melted away. Such a paradigm shift has resulted in a marked improvement in the depth of therapeutic outcomes, and in my clinical skills as well.

The information contained in this piece of dreamwork is indeed very impressive; *take my word for it*! Such material is probably priceless in providing information for the operations of the mind. On the other hand, we still do not seem to really know—speculations aside—*what* it represents, *how* it is put together, and where. The book will cautiously explore these fundamental questions about mental images.

---

[3] Flying birds were frequent oracular occurrences in ancient Greece, and their doing so on the right was often a positive omen.

PART I

Learning the Languages

Chapter 1

Humanity's Search for Mind and the Subject: A Brief Review of the Evolution of Neuropsychobiology

The evolutionary path of humanity is speckled with attempts to experience self-definition, to understand mental phenomena, and to express them in a recognizable language. These attempts to clarify mind and the human subject have not been limited to the personal dimension but have also invested in a major way the suprapersonal—the "divine" being a significant example—by way of myth, science, religion, art, philosophy, and the like. The mode of these expressive efforts has been as varied as the disciplines involved: from the construction of gods to mathematical equations and electrochemical diagrams; and, like the disciplines themselves, these languages often *appeared* to be totally unrelated to each other.

At the individual level, humanity has repeatedly conveyed its concern with an instinctual belief that the subject is not so much a single, unitary phenomenon but rather a composite made up of "parts," of structures that escape the boundaries of conscious awareness. These structures are nevertheless perceived as inner experiences and find consensual validation in the subjective experience of others. In a similar manner humanity has struggled with the *motus cordis*, the moving of the heart, those inner events of affective energy that seem to constantly circumvent the logic of conscious awareness. The symbols and metaphors used have changed throughout cultures and time, but the movements of the heart have remained rather constant and always recognizable in that they evoke a sense of familiarity outside the realm of rational understanding (this language of the heart is the major expressive tool of all genuinely creative artistic endeavors). In a majority of cases the true meaning behind the expressive effort remains invisible and eludes the logically based "reasons" used to explain the observable outcome.

If we look back in time for examples of these efforts to capture the inner structure of the human subject, we may reflect on the elaborate "soul" concept that flourished in ancient Egypt. Rather astonishingly, we find that the individual "psyche" was actually conceptualized as a conglomerate of "spiritual" structures (we would now use the term *psychological structures*[1]): the *Sahu*, a spiritual body image mirroring the physical body, the *Ka*, an abstract personality or individuality with an independent existence, equivalent to the Coptic Κω (double), to the Greek έίδωλον or double image, mental attributes; the *Ba*, or heart-soul, the transcendent aspect of the subject; the *Khaibit*, or shadow of the subject, an entirely independent function counter-pointing the Ka and the Ba and equivalent to the Greek σκια and to the Roman *umbra*; the *Khu* (spirit-soul), another transcendent function; the *Sekhem* (transcendent vital power); the *Ren* (the person's name). Originally the Egyptians considered all these parts as separate from each other in the afterlife, but in later times these concepts became bound together in a form that resembled the subject and included the divine aspect: the *Osiris* of that subject (Budge, 1895/1960).

I have presented in some detail the Egyptian belief in the nonphysical characteristics of a person as an elaborate but by no means exclusive example of the human perception that mind is functionally a complex composite. The visible reason—the religious explanation—may have been incorrect, but this absence of a correct visible reason only puts greater emphasis on the mystery and poignancy of the underlying theme: the search for a way to give expression to the universally felt, complex structure of the psychological subject. While the meaning of this universally felt psychological structure escapes us, its existence stands reaffirmed.

It may be revealing that it took over a millennium after the Egyptians had designed a model of the spiritual subject, for the Greeks across the Mediterranean Sea to discover the human mind in a psychological sense—if we accept the deep analysis of this process conducted by the German classicist Bruno Snell (1896/1982). Through an attentive exploration of the words and notions expressed in Greek literature from Homer to Callimachus—and of how they evolved and changed—Snell depicts the progressive integration of "parts" of the human experience into an emerging concept of self, the movement from mythical to logical thought and the origin of scientific thinking. We can push our review of the emergence and structure of the human subject much further

---

[1] These structures should not be dismissed as curios from the past, but should rather be considered and reflected upon. For example, what caused them to emerge into being in the collective conscious mind of the time? How did they come to exist? Out of what psychological need did they emerge, and what need or value do they imply? They were "felt" images that percolated into consciousness from a subjective "intuition" around some internal tension and that found intersubjective validation. They were as real and gravid of meaning as our most felt beliefs (an echo to the Egyptian metaphor of a "subject-as-Osiris" can still be found in the modern image of the "subject-as-Christ").

back in time, and we will continue to observe the appearance of symbols carrying a meaning different from what they seem to describe.

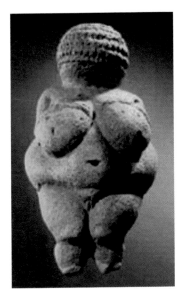

Figure 1-1 represents a famous "Venus," possibly the earliest extant representation of the feminine, dated at approximately 25,000 BCE, a metaphor for sure of the artist's *motus cordis*, but its true meaning is hidden, as it most likely was to the artist too (inside the artist's "heart" some "feminine" element compelled its being captured and made permanent, visible, tangible). Figure 1-2 brings us to an equally remote past, around 20,000 years BCE.

The expression of a different *motus cordis* required here that a human subject crawl literally into the bowels of Earth for almost a mile, through a narrow, twisting natural tunnel, in damp darkness but for some torchlike object; carrying dust pigments of several colors in order to paint on the stones of the walls and roof magnificent herds of buffaloes and horses and deers that 20,000 years later are still moving, at the flicker of lights, along their dimensions of stone.

Figure 1-1: The Venus of Willendorf. Naturhistoisches Museum, Vienna. (Photo by author)

Minds barely at the level of primitive speech, who interpreted the world in a way that is totally hidden to us, went to great lengths and unusual ways in order to express and capture something ineffable (presumably, the place that they chose added a specific implication and represented a needed tool in order

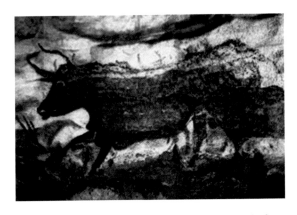

Figure 1-2: Buffalo, Prehistoric cave painting, Perigord. (Photo by author)

to obtain the sought-for outcome) and left a meaning, an obscure message of their thinking processes, of their mental activity, of their systems of values

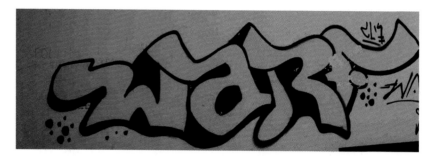

Figure 1-3: Italian graffito. Finale, Italy. (Photo by author)

and beliefs. Did they know what they were actually trying to capture within themselves and express through their paintings? Probably not any more than the Egyptians did with their afterlife metaphors, or the graffito painters of Figure 1-3.

The dynamic experience of the human mind is an intrinsically subjective event of immense proportions, as will be clarified later on in the text, that continues to readjust to evolutionary dynamics, inclusive of culture and civilization; this may explain the difficulty that humanity has faced and continues to face when probing the matter (as I have stated elsewhere [1999] "the subjective mind is a mystery within a mystery.") Furthermore, subjective phenomena have been perceived as not demonstrably physical in nature; they are not quantifiable and usually cannot be replicated. They seem to fall outside the four principles that represent the foundations of scientific materialism.

Objectivism: Empirical facts are testable by empirical methods and verifiable by third-person means.
Monism: We live in one universe made by one kind of stuff that can be described completely by physics.
Reductionism: Macrophenomena are the causal result of microphenomena.
Closure principle: The physical world is causally closed. There are no causal influences on physical events except for other physical events.

This apparently irreducible conflict caused a progressive schism between subjectivity with its psychological language and science in general—specifically neuroscience. In order to hide the lack of fit between the science and the data, (subjective) mental events were "reframed" in objective terms. Behaviorism reduced all subjective mental activity to objective behavior and neuroscience reduced it to objective brain activity (see also Wallace, 2000, p. 24).

Consequently, while the various organizations of mental contents that had so baffled the Egyptians and the Greeks became increasingly integrated into a single psychological construct, the dichotomy between psychology and "recognized" science deepened. The necessarily very brief review that completes this chapter will address the progressive organization of the "I" in psychological terms, and some of the key factors contributing to it. This review retraces in part the path outlined in the excellent work of Australian cultural scientist Nick Mansfield (2000), who traced the relationships during the past 5 centuries between the conceptualization of the subject and the cultural forces that may have contributed to molding the field and the understanding of subjectivity.

The process of differentiation from myth to logic, and the growing reliance on conscious logic as the main field of self-expression and self-understanding, gradually fostered a disconnection between the rational, conscious ego (logos) and the irrational domain of the *motus cordis* (Eros) that had played a central role in the world of myths. At the beginning of this journey the subject (and not necessarily the hero) had been largely an actor of sorts, playing a role imposed by forces well defined as outside the self, usually located in the supra-natural realm of the divine. In the Greek epics about the age of the heroes (reflecting a bronze age palace culture that existed from approximately 1600 BCE to 1200 BCE), and in particular in the works of Homer, we realize that the interest was primarily upon the event itself and its inevitable unfolding. This focus is more recognizable in the Iliad tragedy than in the more recent, romantic *Odyssey* that was possibly written by a different mind from the one who wrote the *Iliad*. In these epics the human beings express the decisions of the gods. Attempts to modify the course of the events are immediately and constantly counteracted by the intervention of a divinity—as in the role of Athena in sealing the fate of Hector, in book 22 of the *Iliad*, when, disguised as Hector's brother, she tricks him to stop his flight and face Achilles and his own death.

Epic, as Snell (1896/1982) aptly remarks, "tells myths, it accepts them as reality and arranges them on two levels, one existing on earth and the other in heaven" (p. 96). In the Greek tragedies of a later era, the focus shifts from the event itself to the human beings and questions the significance of mythical reality. The divine level loses its primacy; mythical reality becomes fundamentally a reality of humanity that involves universal concepts offering definition to particular ones. It is a structure gravid with timeless significance and always susceptible to recurrence.

Beginning with Solon and proceeding through the pre-Socratic and post-Socratic philosophers, to culminate with Plato and Aristotle, the cleavage between mythical and logical thought becomes established; in Snell's words, "mythical thought is closely related to the thinking in images and similes. Psychologically speaking, both differ from logical thought in that the latter searches and labors while the figures of myth and the images of the similes burst fully-shaped upon the imagination" (1896/1982, p. 224).

Soul is defined by Aristotle as the perfect realization of a natural body (1936/1986, par. 402–412). There is a close connection between psychological states and physiological processes. The Latin expression "mens sana in corpore sano" (a healthy mind in a healthy body) will reflect this Aristotelian principle throughout the following 2 millennia. Body and soul are a single system, in a similar relation to each other as the wax and an impression stamped on it. However, the soul—or mind—is not simply the product of the physiological conditions of the body, but is the *truth* of the body, the substance that permits the meaningful realization of all bodily conditions. Aristotle describes "faculties" as parts of the mind and the expression of different stages in biological development: nutrition (plant kingdom), movement (animal kingdom), and reason (peculiar to humans) organized hierarchically, with the higher one including the lower. The mind, although made of these "parts," is conceptualized as intrinsically unitary, and Aristotle therefore rejects Plato's position that the mind can desire with one part and simultaneously feel anger with another part. Aristotelian thinking came also to represent the first organized system of scientific thought and continues to constitute the substrate of Western natural science.

The process of separating the rational mind from the mythical/irrational— that became gradually tinted with "dark" characteristics, as pagan, magical, inferior functions, animal traits, and the like and that had formed the basis of Aristotle's dichotomy of the soul—continued with Christianity, that perfected the schism by externalizing much of Eros into the "non-God" side of evil and Satan. The psychological dichotomy of the subject into a conscious, rational-good side and an unconscious, irrational-bad one affected also the orientation of modern science. "What we really believe to be true will invariably influence what we believe to be of value; conversely, all of us, including scientists, seek to understand those aspects of reality that we value. Thus, the scientific worldview has been generated by the kinds of values and ideals held by the scientists. The mutual interdependence of values and beliefs is inescapable" (Wallace, 2000, p. 7).

The hypertrophic importance given during the past 400 years to a specific type of consciousness (see Chapter 5) became fully defined in the works of René Descartes (1596–1650) and permeated that period of human cultural development that became known as the Enlightenment and still pervades modern Western institutions. Descartes introduced into the scientific process the equation of consciousness equal to conscious awareness, or what neuro-scientist Gerald Edelman (1992) calls "higher order consciousness" or "conscious of being conscious" (p. 112). Presumably this is the state in which intellect and reason reside, and the Cartesian message proclaimed reason as the highest evolutionary achievement, which constitutes the quintessence of the human subject, separating humanity from all other biological organisms.

Consequently, conscious awareness has become immensely seductive. It is a very powerful tool, but it has its limitations and its dangers, as I will discuss.

The Cartesian cogito ergo sum dictates also that rational thinking is equivalent to essence: conscious awareness becomes the mode of being of what has been (erroneously) called the self, but actually in psychological terms is only the ego.[2] For Descartes the subject is therefore a clearly defined unit fully contained in its own state of consciousness.

The Cartesian "emphasis on the conscious as the defining faculty of the self" (Mansfield, 2000, p. 18) became strengthened approximately a century later by the work of Immanuel Kant (1724–1804) who in his *Critique* of *Pure Reason* stated that the very *formation* of the self requires consciousness. "For Kant, subjectivity can only have content through awareness of the world" (Mansfield, 2000, p. 19). Kant's contemporary Jean-Jacques Rousseau differs from the two previous thinkers in that he considers all individual experiences, and not only reason and intellect, as expressions of the subject and important in their totality in order to acquire self-knowledge and self-understanding. As Mansfield (2000) notes, Rousseau and Kant best exemplify "the contradiction between the attempt to grasp the individual experience as a totality and the belief that its essence and truth are to be found in conscious processes" alone (p. 20). Such contradiction is still alive today and we will encounter it over and over.

The common position of the entire Enlightenment movement viewed the self (or, more precisely, the ego) "as a completely self-contained being that develops in the world as an expression of its own unique essence" (Mansfield, 2000, p. 13). With this postulation humanity appears to have traveled a long way, almost swinging to the opposite pole from the Greek hero figure, who was largely an expression of divine will. And perhaps it has tried to push even further, toward complete liberation from any other root than its own and its "intelligence," to a position of never before reached hubris (while the Greek gods used men to solve their own squabbles, modern man uses the gods to justify prevailing over the "Other"). We may be facing now the retribution for such arrogance, as we stand, psychologically alone, disconnected from an intrinsic spiritual dimension by the barrier of the organized, enlightened religious systems of our time, whose symbols have been flattened out, corroded by time, and lost meaning; while the barrier of "pure reason" separates us from the potential of our great psychic depth.

However, with the Freudian breakthrough things began to change. The unconscious dimension of the self was rediscovered and given serious attention

---

[2] These two incorrect equations (consciousness = conscious awareness and self/subject = ego) have permeated all nonpsychological scientific approaches to mind, and some of the psychological too, as behaviorism and ego/cognitive psychology.

by the different schools that branched out of Freud's teachings; its attributes became progressively less demonized and its fundamental influence, even upon reason and logic, was again recognized. The "Freudian revolution" had been preannounced by a growing concern with the splintered self. Works of literature tried to deal with the internal split and Mansfield (2000) accurately indicates Mary Shelley's *Frankenstein* (1818), Robert Louis Stevenson's *The Strange Case of Doctor Jekyll and Mr. Hyde* (1886), and Dostoyevsky's *The Double* (1846/1958) as examples of the divided self before Freud. These three works show in a quite dramatic way the process that will culminate in the emergence of the psychoanalytic movements.

In *Frankenstein* we still observe a full externalization of the "irrational" and demonic inside of us into the primal "monster." As the two entities or polarities cannot be contained within the same psychic space, what follows is the inevitable shared annihilation of both.

In *Dr. Jekyll and Mr. Hyde* the split has now moved within the subject but the two psychic structures are still profoundly different and alien to each other; the transformation is triggered by an external factor that deranges the "legitimate" self; "badness" is not necessarily intrinsic but rather caused by "the potion" of evil, by tampering with the mind.

The *Double*, on the contrary, is a reassessment of the hero's inner self. Although the metaphor is played out through an external, never-before met "twin," actually the subject has to confront unrecognized aspects of the self. Furthermore, these aspects are not any more "irrational" and primitive, although they might be dark and unpalatable to the ego.

The stage was set for the emergence of psychoanalytic research on these unconscious aspects of the subject and their role in and weight upon the entire organization of mind. With the introduction of the unconscious as a main system in the regulation of mental functions Freud overthrew the Cartesian consciousness, until this was reintroduced in American psychiatry by ego psychology.

The entire psychoanalytic family attempts to define the subject as an entity, even if the roots to such entity may be differently identified in the different theories that branched out of the Freudian position. For all these theories, the subject is intrinsically real and distinct from the world, although imbedded in it.

To Freudian psychoanalysis, the dominant relationships that contribute to subjectivity are family relationships defined in terms of gender and sexuality. Therefore, the Freudian culture considers the subject as evolving out of neurobiology ("anatomy is destiny"). Key factors to subjectivity are the gender relations and sexual identifications of the child, the prototypical child being the male one, and the point of reference being the penis of the father. It is first a theory of masculinity: a phallocentric and phallocratic system that mars the woman's psychological development with a "lack," which in turn is responsible for the woman subject being less able to fit into societal norm.

Another school of significant interest in the context of this discussion is the one organized around the findings of Freud's once favored pupil, Carl Jung. These two schools, and their respective derivatives, differ from each other primarily in the choice and the significance of the relationships that form the human subject. Although still gender biased, the Jungian school minimized the importance of infantile sexuality and introduced a drastically different, expanded idea of the unconscious populated by ancient ("archetypal") systems or instincts that represent the templates of basic mental organizations (as maternity/matriarchy and paternity/patriarchy, divinity, selfhood, gender, life roles, and the like) as they were laid down at the dawn of humanity and were subsequently molded by culture. These instinctual inherited fields of organizing energy—each one containing its own polarity of opposing manifestations— can become differentially activated as the subject experiences life and its relationships. While subjectivity for Freud reflected the primary relationship with the genital father, the Jungian subject reflects the complex of relationships between the individual experience and these collective blueprints as they may be played out in the world of external objects.

The self represents the theater, the center of this process as well as its full expression, and its domain is primarily unconscious. The ego continues to represent, as in the Freudian organization of psyche, that function of the subject invested with conscious awareness. The drama is not anymore played between the emerging subject and the internalized meaning of the penis of the father; rather, it is played between the emerging self and the dictates of these systems that represent the collective "legacy" of the species and need to be reorganized and reframed in terms of individual autonomy. The Jungian school dusted off and reintroduced the mythical language in the context of this struggle between the individual and the legacy of our past: the subject is seen as a hero of sorts involved in a personal journey through life, a journey constellated by recognizable mythical patterns and images.

The phallocratic stance of Freudian theory generated a significant amount of critical reframing by the feminist psychoanalysts. In general (paraphrasing Mansfield, 2000, p. 73), feminism argues simply that in patriarchal cultures gender roles are imposed on nature, not derived from it. In reality, the opposite is true: biology (sex) comes first, and then culture (gender) (Mansfield, 2000, p. 73). The positions of Donna Haraway (1991), Julia Kristeva (1982), and Jessica Benjamin (1998) will be presented later on, in different contexts.

Luce Irigaray (1980) contrasts a plural and dynamic feminine genital conformation (and a culture not of the visible but of the tangible and continuous) with the phallomorphic masculine focus on the singular and the unified. The result is a complex and fluid subjectivity. "The feminine does not insist on a strict dividing line between the self and what is outside of it (the other)" (Mansfield, 2000, p. 72). We will encounter again this stance in the work of Benjamin, and evaluate its relevance to the concept of intersubjectivity. Judith Butler (1993) argues that gender subjectivity is not an intrinsic event, but rather a product of culture, and it comes first, constructing nature in its own image. The tyranny of gender over social behavior is quite evident and affects every aspect of social life. By suggesting that gender may be more a product of the social system than an intrinsic characteristic of the subject she aligns herself with the antisubjective position. Mansfield, in tracing the anti-subjective movement, compares those theories that try to define the subject as an entity in its own right with theories that question the intrinsic reality of the subject and challenge the self/object demarcation, or boundary, but see any definition of subjectivity as the product of power and culture.

For Michel Foucault (1980), Rousseau's self-sufficient individual is an illusion. The individual is an effect of power (specific bodies, gestures, discourses, desires are selected by power) and at the same time it is the element of its articulation, the vehicle of power. The dominant relationships that contribute to subjectivity "are the broad relationships of power and subordination that are present everywhere in all societies" (Mansfield, 2000, p. 32). "The subject does not exist as a naturally occurring entity, but is contrived by the double work of power and knowledge to maximize the operation of both" (Mansfield, 2000, p. 72).

It is interesting to recall that Foucault's theory was also promulgated, independently, by Marxist philosopher Louis Althusser (1971) who postulated that ideology needs subjectivity. The subject exists for the system that needs it. Subjectivity is the type of being one becomes as one fits into the needs of the (capitalist) state (Mansfield, 2000, p. 53). This is a very ancient theme indeed, reformulated in rational, Cartesian terms! Another version of Foucault's position was that of the gods, from the Egyptian Kephera to the Sumerian Enki and the Indian Prajapati, and even the Christian God. They all found themselves needing self-actualization and therefore created humanity, "in their similitude," in order to clarify their own existence and meaning.

Concomitantly with the preoccupation for its psychic attributes, humanity searched also for a deeper understanding of the body and for the physical site of mind. The birth of neuroscience can also be traced back to ancient Egypt. Around 1700 BCE, while the concepts of Ka (and Ba, and Khu) were depicted in the sacred texts, the hieroglyphic symbol 𓄏𓊪𓏤 for brain found its first known appearance in the Edwin Smith papyrus (also known as the surgical papyrus) that describes several anatomical characteristics of the central nervous system.

One has to wait 1000 years before a similar scientific interest in the brain emerges on the other side of the Mediterranean; Hippocrates (460–379 BCE) relates epilepsy to brain dysfunction and discusses his belief that mental processes are located in the brain. Plato has the same idea, while Aristotle will dissent and locate mental functions in the heart.

Science has then to wait 1½ millennia, after Galen's (170 CE) position that the brain is the source of perception and voluntary motion as well as the center of rational thought. Only in the 16th century, with the great anatomists Leonardo Da Vinci, Vesalius, Falloppio, Eustachio, Varolio, and Piccolomini among others, did organized interest in neuroanatomy and neuroscience emerge from the Dark Ages.

The study of brain structure acquired further impetus with the advent of the microscope (Janssen, 1590), which opened previously inconceivable vistas and moved observation to the cellular level.

In the 19th century, following Galvani's, Volta's, and Bell's breakthroughs in electrical manipulation, neuroscience added the dimension of neuroelectrophysiology to the study of static structures or experimentation on animals (living human specimens had not been officially available for dissection since the end of the Ptolemaic period in Alexandria). The dynamic studies on discrete circuits and functions of the brain flourished, as did the "new" discipline of psychology: William James published *Principles of Psychology* in 1890; in 1900 Freud published *The Interpretation of Dreams* and almost simultaneously, neuroelectrophysiologist Sherrington attempted a metaphoric integration of brain and mind in his work *Man on His Nature* (1940–1951). "The brain is waking and with it the mind is returning. It is as if the Milky Way entered upon some cosmic dance. Swiftly the head mass becomes an enchanted loom where millions of flashing shuttles weave a dissolving pattern, always a meaningful pattern though never an abiding one; a shifting of subpatterns" (Sherrington, 1940/1951, p. 15).

From the perspective of cognitive neuroscience one of the next most significant works is possibly *The Organization of Behavior: A Neuropsychological Theory* by Donald O. Hebb (1949). His introduction into modern neuroscience of the concepts of *assemblies of neurons* and of *synaptic strengthening* through joint activation came to represent two cardinal foundations for all modern research (see Chapter 3 for further discussion). The evolution of computers introduced yet another significant approach to the search for greater understanding of brain function. As Haykin states in his book (1994), "*Neural Networks*, or artificial neural networks to be more precise, represent an emerging technology rooted in many disciplines" (p. v). "Work on artificial neural networks... has been motivated right from its inception by the recognition that the brain computes in an entirely different way from the conventional digital computer.... The brain is a highly *complex, nonlinear, and parallel computer* (information-processing system)" (p. 1). A recent and fascinating set of tools that aid us in the study of the brain during its diverse functions is offered by the field of radio imaging: the various techniques used to visualize central nervous system dynamics have opened breathtaking windows into the secrets of this stunning organ. In spite of all these tools, mind continues to elude. Neuroscientist Damasio (1999) states that "There is a mystery, however, regarding how images emerge from neural patterns. How a neural pattern becomes an image is a problem that neurobiology has not yet resolved" (Damasio, 1999, p. 322).

Chapter 2

AN "IDEOGRAPHIC," SUPRAPERSONAL LANGUAGE OF RULES AND UNIVERSAL SYMBOLS: ALWYN SCOTT AND NONLINEAR DYNAMICS

The brain contains 100 billion neurons, of which 10 to 30 billion are in the cerebral cortex. There are an average of 10,000 to 100,000 synapses per neuron, accounting for 1 million billion connections. A conservative estimate of the number of ideas or concepts that a neo-cortex can store in the form of cell assemblies is at least equal to 10^{10} (10 billion) (Scott, 2002, p. 276).[1] As this is also the number of seconds in 300 years, it seems ample for the memories that we gather in the course of a normal life. However, this number (10^{10}) is far less than the number of possible ways that the neocortex can be organized.[2] The number of possible neural circuits, or mental states, or individual minds, which could be constructed from all the possible dynamic patterns among the assemblies is at least as large as

$$10^{10^{17}}.$$

In order to give some perspective to this number,[3] recall that physicist Walter Elsasser (1998) defined any finite number greater than 10^{110} as an

---

[1] This is a large but still a finite number. "Because the number of neurons in the neocortex is 10^{10} and a typical cell assembly might involve (say) 10^4 neurons, some mistakenly suppose that the number of possible assemblies is only 10^6 (John Eccles made this mistake). Confusion arises because one neuron can participate in more than one assembly" (Scott, personal communication).

[2] "One way to see this is that two people with the same 10^{10} assemblies would still have them organized (or interrelated) differently. Upon seeing the color red, one person might think of an apple, another a sunset, another his lover's dress, and so on" (Scott, personal communication). Such reorganization of neural connectivity is ongoing also *in the same brain, with every thought or experience we have.*

[3] Scott (1995, p. 213); Edelman and Tononi (2000, p. 38). This is a hyperimmense number.

"immense number."[4] What was his motivation? As 10^{80} is about equal to the atomic mass of the universe (number of protons in the universe) and 10^{30} is the age of the universe in picoseconds (the basic time unit of chemical dynamics), it is not possible to realize all examples of an immense number of possibilities. The number of possible protein molecules, for example, is immense, so all possible proteins have not and never will be realized.

The number expressed above is a conservative lower bound on the number of possible brains, and it is much, much larger than Elsasser's immense number (actually, it is the immense number multiplied by itself 10,000 trillion times; Scott, 1995, p. 213). Therefore the complexity of the structural organization that forms the foundation to mind can be described as hyperimmense and justifies the opinion of many scientists that the brain is the most complicated known physical structure in the entire universe and that its connectivity, dynamics, and ways it relates to the body and to the world are like nothing else science has ever encountered. This level of complexity and versatility requires operational laws that allow for noncomputational systems and the necessity for such requirement is evident when one considers that, to begin with, the billions of connections are not exactly replicated in every brain: no two brains are identical, even for identical twins. The microscopic variability at the level of the finest ramifications of neurons is immense, so that each brain presents a substantially unique synaptic architecture. Furthermore, each brain has a unique developmental and experiential history that is ever-changing, so that from day to day the synaptic connectivity in the same brain is subject to changes. Also, the relationship between cause and effect in the biological world is not that clear and linear. Finally, the brain is presented with complex series of signals, profoundly different from the binary signals of a computer language and carrying a different meaning, or value, from one subject to the other and even within the same brain, in response to different subtle experiences with reality. Therefore their impact on synaptic dynamics is unpredictable and unreplicable.

In the opinion of mathematician Roger Penrose (1994), "within the strait-jacket of an entirely computational physics ... there can be no scientific role for intentionality and subjective experience" (p. 420). This view, shared by a score of neuroscientists, urges for the identification of a system of universal operational laws that could apply to the biological organism and to the operations of the brain.

Table 2-1 compares three sets of physics as they might pertain to the dynamics of the mind.

---

[4] The number of particles (mass) of the universe is about 10^{80}. The age of the universe (20 billion years) in units of picoseconds (10^{-12} seconds) is about 10^{30}. Their product is roughly equal to 10^{110}.

Table 2-1: Core characteristics of three sets of physics.

Linear physics	Nonlinear physics	Quantum physics
Deterministic: B will always follow A	Acausal: The relationship between cause and effect is obscure	Indeterminate: Collapse is uncertain because it is radically contingent
Reductionistic: C is always = B+A)	Emergent: The whole is greater than the sum of its parts	Emergent: C is different than A+B
Atomistic: The world ultimately consists of separate bits that cannot form creative relationships The physics of "either/or"	Holistic: At each level of description additional entities emerge that cannot be reduced to more simple descriptions Biological and cognitive sciences are conceptually unbounded	Holistic: Separateness is at best an approximation The physics of "both/and"

1. Newtonian or classical, linear physics has been the very foundation of scientific materialism and with its strict predictability and algorithmic nature it has been very beneficial to physical science and to an understanding of the physical world. However, the same characteristics make it unfit to support inherently noncomputable models of brain function.

2. Quantum mechanics has raised serious attention among scholars, and models of a quantal mind had produced high expectations. John Eccles (1991), Roger Penrose, and Stuart Hameroff (1998) have been among the most significant exponents of this position. Today, the interest in a quantal mind has dimmed due to the lack of supporting evidence against the insurmountable obstacles to meaningful quantal states in the biological organism. Interest has moved back from esoteric systems of physics to models that are more anchored to classical reality and yet allow for a noncomputational approach to brain function and may permit us to understand the emergence of mental events.

3. Nonlinear dynamics appears to be such a system. It counterpoints the linear systems that have been favored by physical scientists because "a complex cause can be expressed as a convenient sum of single components, and the combined effect is the sum of the effects from each component of the total cause" (Scott, 1995, p. 189). Neuroscientist and mathematician Alwyn Scott is a major exponent of this mathematical language that describes universals, among which the biological domain and therefore the brain are included. In

presenting this language I will therefore stay as close as possible to his images and concepts.[5]

In mathematics the term *nonlinear* is defined in the context of the relationships between cause and effects (Scott, 2002, p. 300). Suppose that a series of experiments conducted on a certain system shows that cause $C1$ gives rise to effect $E1$ and that cause $C2$ gives rise to effect $E2$; the system under observation will be linear if:

$$C(1) + C(2) \text{ causes } E(1) + E(2).$$

The system will be nonlinear if:

$$C(1) + C(2) \text{ does not cause } E(1) + E(2).$$

In nature and in all biological organisms most systems are nonlinear and generally the effect from the sum of two causes is not equal to the sum of the individual effects. As a very simplified example, if the release of neurotransmitter (A) causes the firing of neuron (Y) and the release of neurotransmitter (B) causes the firing of neuron (X), then:

- the system will be linear if the simultaneous release of $(A) + (B)$ causes the firing of (Y) and (X) only.
- The system will be nonlinear if the simultaneous release of the two neurotransmitters will cause something different than the exclusive firing of (Y) and (X).

The equation $(C1 + C2) \neq (E1 + E2)$, which can be verbalized as *the whole is not equal to the sum of its parts,* constitutes the most fundamental tenet of nonlinear dynamics and a radical departure from linear science.

Nonlinearity is not a convenient situation for the researcher because it implies rather untidy conditions, where multiple causes interact among themselves rather than proceeding in a sequential predictable fashion; therefore they allow for many more outcomes than the anticipated ones, and in so doing confound the constructionist.

However, for these very reasons nonlinearity plays a key role in the course of biological evolution. Nonlinear emergence has a clear relationship with *positive feedback*, which happens whenever phenomenon (A) causes (B) but (B) in its turn causes (A). A closed causal loop operates between the two phenomena

---

[5] For an overview of the role that nonlinear dynamics may play in trying to understand "the collective dynamics of billions of interconnected neurons in the brain" see also Glanz (1997).

which is self-sustaining because (*A*) causes enough (*B*) to support the original level of (*A*) and vice versa. The loop could be represented as:

These self-sustaining loops lead directly to the phenomenon of emergence. Out of their interactive dynamics something new appears. Scott uses as an example the loop between the burning wick of a candle that by generating heat causes the melting of the wax, which in turn sustains the burning of the wick. The emergent phenomenon out of the dynamics of this loop—or level of events—is the flame itself.

Another illustration of a positive feedback, self-sustaining loop is depicted in Figure 2-1 (adapted from Goldstein and Volkow, 2002).

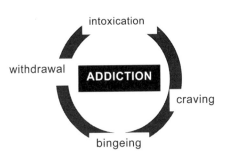

Figure 2-1: Positive loop in drug addiction. Rita Z. Goldstein and Nora D. Volkow, "Drug Addiction and Its Underlying Neurobiological Basis: Neuroimaging Evidence for the Involvement of the Frontal Cortex," *American J. Psychiatry*, Oct. 2002; 159:1643–1652. Figure 1. (Reprinted by permission.)

Four clusters of phenomena—each already the expression of lower level dynamics—are interactive in a self-supporting loop. Out of these dynamic interactions a new, higher-level outcome emerges; *addiction*; its dynamics will interact with other higher-level phenomena (psychological, social, legal, medical, financial) and out of these interactions still other outcomes will emerge. Among the most salient emergent outcomes Scott includes a nerve impulse, a storm, a city, living organisms, perhaps even mind.

The variables that participate in the ultimate definition of the outcome define the *phase space* for that particular process. The phase space, a term that indicates the space that could contain all the possible combinations, is a system of coordinates that define each possible state of the system.

Therefore, a phase space can be very complicated, and it may be compounded by the presence of *attractors*, or conditions that impose a specific, "local" directional weight.

As a simplistic example, imagine a bee buzzing around. The three-dimensional space is the phase space for the bee's flight (actually, the space is four-dimensional because it involves time also). If a bit of sugar is now located somewhere in the phase space, the random flight of the insect will begin to show a change in pattern and eventually the bee will zoom to the sugar. The sugar is a local attractor (naturally, this specific attractor will not have any effect—or a different one—if it is imbedded in the phase space of a cat).

New dynamic entities stem from the presence of these closed causal loops. The nonlinear causal dynamics operating at each level of description generate emergent structures, and nonlinear interactions among these structures provide a basis for the dynamics of the next higher level.

Are these systems of recursive dynamics an inherent aspect of life or are they simply another metaphor without substance? In other words, are they necessary to explain upper level phenomena, or could these levels be derived from lower level ones in a linear fashion, without the need for positive feedback and closed loops phenomena? As Scott points out, this consideration brings into the discussion the theory of *reductionism*, which has provided a very successful approach to the understanding of the natural world and includes three steps:

1. *Analysis*: The investigator who needs to explain a higher-level phenomenon breaks it down into "components" that can then be separately investigated.
2. *Theoretical formulation*: The investigator develops a theory of how these "components" interact by means of empirical observations and of imagination.
3. *Synthesis*: The investigator explains the higher-level phenomenon in concordance with the theory.

Reductionism postulates that all natural phenomena can be explained in this way. Some of the critics of the reductionistic philosophy sustain that some natural phenomena, such as life itself, cannot be completely described in terms of lower-level entities. This position takes two forms: on one side, *substance dualists* argue that substantial aspects of the physical world do not have a *physical basis*. The more restrained, subdued *property* dualists share the opinion that all aspects of the natural world have a *physical basis*, but assert that some aspects of the physical world cannot be understood in terms of atomic or molecular dynamics.

To the critics of reductionism Scott (2002) proposes as a common foundation that "all natural phenomena *supervene* on the physical in the following sense. If the constituent matter is removed the phenomenon in question disappears" (p. 295). This position is known as *physicalism*. (The position carries also for the phenomenon of life: if the atoms are gradually removed from a biological organism, it will eventually die.)

Reductive physicalism is a serious position, schematically illustrated in Figure 2-2. In this example a higher-level phenomenon M_1 is supported by lower-level physical properties P_1. If the properties P_1 are removed the phenomenon M_1 eventually disappears. The same can be expected from the relationship between P_2 and M_2.

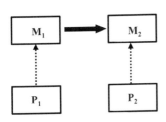

Figure 2-2: The causal interaction of higher-level phenomena (M_1 and M_2) that supervene on lower-level properties (P_1 and P_2) (adapted from Scott, 2002).

Furthermore, if observation at the upper level indicates a causal relationship between M_1 and M_2, one can infer that the same causal relationship is present also between P_1 and P_2 "which is a formulation of the upper-level causality in terms of the lower-level properties" (Scott, 2002, p. 296).

The upward-directed arrows can be formulated at every level of description, showing the direction of reductive implication. "These arrows ultimately emanate from the most fundamental element of physical reality (nowadays known as the 'Higgs boson')" (Scott, 2002, p. 296). Such a viewpoint implies that although it may be impractical or currently impossible to describe the dynamics of a biological organism in terms of the fundamental fields and particles of physics, nevertheless it could be done, at least in principle.

However, the computable, unidirectional approach of reductionistic physicalism, which has been very appropriate to the physical sciences, has shown problems when applied to the biological world. First of all, reductionism does not automatically imply (re) constructionism: physicist Philip Anderson (1972) states that "the ability to reduce everything to simple fundamental laws does not imply the ability to start from those laws and reconstruct the universe" (p. 394).[6] Furthermore, the constructionist hypothesis breaks down when confronted with the scale and the complexity inherent to biological structures. As Scott suggests, one may consider the proteins: these are strings

---

[6] One is reminded of Ms. Tangerine's search for what makes an artwork (Pratchett, 2001):

> The frame that once had been (the painting of) Wagon Stuck in River was leaning against a wall in front of her. It was empty. The bare canvas was neatly rolled beside it. In front of the frame, carefully heaped in order of size, were piles of pigments. Several dozen Auditors were breaking these down into their component molecules. "Still nothing?" she said, striding along the line. "No, Miss Tangerine. Only known molecules and atoms so far." said an Auditor, its voice shaking slightly. "Well... is it something to do with the proportions? The balance of molecules? The basic geometry?" "We are continuing to look ..." "Go on with it!" (p. 262)

of the 20 available aminoacids in various combinations and patterns, and each protein on the average contains around 200 of them. Therefore the number of possible proteins is 20^{200}, which is significantly greater than the immense number of Elsasser. Given that the number of particles in the entire universe is 10^{80}, it follows that "all the matter of the myriad galaxies falls far short of that required to construct but one example of each possible protein molecule. Through the eons of life on Earth most of the possible proteins have never been constructed and never will be" (Scott, 2002, p. 297). All the proteins known to us were selected in the course of evolution through a succession of historical accidents that are *consistent with but not governed by the laws of physics and chemistry.*

The protein state of affairs repeats itself at all levels of the biological hierarchy. The possible number of new entities that can emerge from each level—to form the dynamics for the phenomena at the next level—is immense, "suggesting that happenstance, rather than basic laws of physics, guides important aspects of the evolutionary process" (Scott, 2002, p. 298).

Research in biological science is therefore radically different from research in physics, because in physics repeated experiments can be conducted on identical sets and therefore the scientist can establish precise laws. In biology, on the contrary, the subsets are heterogeneous because of the immense number of possible manifestations that characterize a particular class of phenomena. At best the biological and social scientists can identify only probabilistic rules of conduct for that specific category of phenomena. To conclude, the debate between linearity and nonlinearity indicates that the latter is the approach that best fits the complexity of the biological world, or life.

Earlier on we saw that the term *nonlinear* refers to the relationships between cause and effect. Aristotle (384–322 BCE) made the development of potentiality to actuality one of the most important aspects of his philosophy (it was intended to solve the difficulties which earlier thinkers had raised with reference to the beginnings of existence and the relations of the one and the many). The actual versus potential state of things is explained in terms of the causes that act on things. In the Aristotelian model there are four causes:

1. Material cause, or the elements out of which an object is created;
2. Efficient cause, or the means by which it is created;
3. Formal cause, or the expression of what it is;
4. Final cause, or the end for which it is.

Aristotle's famous example is that of a bronze statue. Its material cause is the bronze itself. Its efficient cause is the sculptor, insofar has he forces the bronze into shape. The formal cause is the idea of the completed statue. The final cause is the idea of the statue as it prompts the sculptor to act on the bronze. For Aristotle, the final cause is internal to the nature of the object itself, and not something we subjectively impose on it. As an example of joint causality in the biological domain Scott returns to the proteins. In the building of a protein molecule the density and variety of aminoacids represent the material cause; the DNA code is the formal cause; the electrostatic and valence forces are the efficient cause (the final cause is hidden).

The most immediate problems that are encountered in applying these concepts to mental events are the definition of material causes and the complexity of efficient causes (as the value systems that will be described in the next chapter), whether they are sufficient to cause a specific mental event, or how much they may participate in such event.

A more general problem is rooted in the direction of causality. In reductionism causality—specifically material and efficient causes—always acts "upwards," from lower levels to higher levels. However, in the biological world one is faced with downward causation, in which variables at the upper level of a hierarchy can place constraints on the dynamics at lower levels and on the expression of the outcome (formal causality). An interesting example may be observed within the context of the intriguing phenomenon of antler shedding among deers. If an alpha male loses a fight for dominance, on the following season his new antlers will be less perfect than the previous ones. The loss of the fight is an unpredictable outcome, not infrequently due to happenstance, such as stepping in a mole burrow with momentary loss of proper position. Still, the loss in social status seems to trigger a downward cascade of neurohormonal reactions that carries through to the following season!

Similarly, a psychological attraction triggered by psychoemotional memories of the person's set of previous interpersonal experiences and specific value systems will modify patterns of neurotransmission and neuromodulation eventuating in the distinctly different mental state and behavior generally named "falling in love" (Marazziti, 2002) or "jealousy". Downward causation does not fit the reductionistic linear model and yet it represents a common phenomenon in the *biological* hierarchy:

Table 2-2: Schematic diagram of the biological hierarchy (Scott, 2002, p. 294).

Biosphere
Species
Organisms
Cells
Processes of replication
Genetic transcription
Biochemical cycles
Molecules

To conclude:

- Self-perpetuating closed causal loops (downward causation) explain much of the biological and human dynamics under physiological as well as pathological conditions.
- The concept of phase space is quite fitting to mental phenomena; indeed, it would be correct to conceptualize the imbedded knowledge of a particular mind as the phase space in the cognitive hierarchy:

Table 2-3: Schematic diagram of the cognitive hierarchy (Scott, 2002, p. 294).

Human cultures
Phase sequence[7]
Complex assemblies
Assemblies of assemblies of assemblies
Assemblies of assemblies
Assemblies of neurons
Neurons
Nerve impulses
Nerve membranes
Membrane proteins
Molecules

In strictly scientific terms this space is too intricate to be represented with any accuracy. We have seen how complex the neuronal phase space is: the space that could contain all the dimensions of neuronal variability and connectivity has been calculated as representing about 100 trillion variables. This phase space (a very large, but finite space) will represent the higher-order assemblies that have actually developed (the ideas that have been thought and that can be viewed as real objects). To this space we have to add all those thoughts that may emerge at any instant as recursive loops with, among others, the upper hierarchical levels of social order and culture (with their own intricate dimensions and combinations). This phase space—what Scott defines as the *dimension of creativity*—is hyperimmense in comparison to the phase space dimension of the cortical neurons.

Even if scientifically uncontainable at the present time, when taken in an illustrative sense these concepts may already offer an invaluable dimension

---

[7] By the term *phase sequence* Hebb implied a thought process in which each assembly action may be aroused by a preceding assembly, a sensory event, or, normally, by both. The central facilitation from one of these activities on the next is the prototype of "attention".

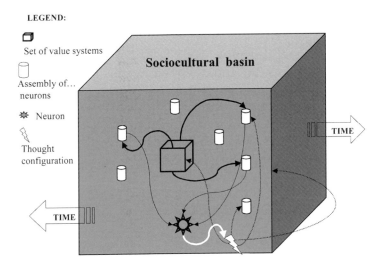

Figure 2-3: Phase space of a mental event (see text for explanation).

to a schematic understanding of mind, as Figure 2-3 indicates. The diagram in Figure 2-3 represents a set of value systems $\Box$, such as the phallocentric patriarchal one described in Chapter 1 and resulting out of the interaction between epigenetic, individualized experiences and "inherited"[8] collective predispositions. This set acts as a local attractor imbedded in the sociocultural basin (consider, for instance, such subsets of Western European culture as the North American or the North European, or orthodox Muslim cultural sects as the Taliban, or yet different systems such as the South African) of a hypothetical mind.

Such an attractor would pose specific constraints upon selected cognitive assemblies $\Box$ (as gender, gender relatedness, contrasexual[9]), which in their turn would establish their own constraints on the electrochemical processes and

---

[8] I do not know how these programs are transcribed from one generation to the next, unless one agrees with Terry Pratchett (2001, p. 72). "Some genetics are passed on via the soul." Biologist Richard Dawkins (1976) introduced the term memes to indicate "a new replicator, a unit of cultural transmission, or a unit of imitation" (p. 192). These replicators deal with elements of human culture and "propagate themselves in the meme pool by leaping from brain to brain via a process which, in the broad sense, can be called imitation. Examples of memes are tunes, ideas, catch-phrases, clothes fashions . . ." (p. 192). He also states that "memes should be regarded as living structures, not just metaphorically but technically" (p. 192) and reports how neuroscientist Juan Delius of the University of Konstanz published a detailed picture of what the neuronal hardware of a meme might look like (p. 323).

[9] The term indicates the inner representations of the opposite sex and the values attached to such components of the self.

synaptic patterns of particular neuronal dynamics and eventuate in a specific thought configuration.[10]

This thought is most likely to act in the context of "internal" self-sustaining positive feedback loops with various cognitive assemblies and with the value system, and even in the context of "external" similar loops with the social structure and the culture, and all their intricate dimensions and combinations. The diagram posits also a *bidirectional* time dimension. The time coordinate is an area out of my league; its placid unidirectional flow got shook-up by relativity and the paradoxes of quantal phenomena; I will leave the scientific details on this bidirectionality to others better qualified to discuss it (see also Scott, 2002, p. 301). However, therapists will not fail to recognize the weird connections between time and the phenomena of developmental regression of the self that occur from the activation in the "present" of "conflicts" that actually are located in the "past" direction of time; or with the reframing of events in the "past" from interventions and insights occurring in the "present."

I will return to Figure 2-3 in later chapters. At this point it suffices to illustrate how the language of nonlinear dynamics—that formulates universal rules for the biological domain—not only contributes to a multidimensional understanding of the mind of humans, but indeed offers the rules and the foundations that support its very existence.

---

[10] I admit my own vagueness about this term. A thought is both a set of electrochemical processes and specific synaptic arrangements and a mental event: Voltaire defines it as "an image that paints itself upon my brain" and I will leave it at that. The existence of thought is not under discussion here, so the language chosen to define the phenomenon is of relative importance at this point.

Chapter 3

A "DEMOTIC," FIRST-PERSON LANGUAGE OF THE INDIVIDUAL AND THE SOCIAL SYSTEM: APULEIUS AND THE MYTH OF PSYCHE

Despite the skittish attitude that modern neuroscience has toward the scientific value of metaphors, the human mind thrives on images and symbols and myths. As Campbell (1973) noted: "It has always been the prime function of mythology and rite to supply the symbols that carry the human spirit forward, in counteraction to those other constant human fantasies that tend to tie it back" (p. 11). The present worldwide investment in the great myths of the major religions is a fitting example. According to Alan Wallace (2000), "between 70 and 90 percent of all Americans believe in a personal God, 80 percent believe in angels ... and only 9 percent believe that God had no part in human development ... from less advanced forms of life. Moreover, 40 percent of the American scientists polled acknowledged their belief in a personal God to whom they can pray, which is roughly the same percentage as a poll taken a century ago" (p. 6).

In the same vein, and talking about mythical figures, in all the major current monotheistic (and patriarchal) societies God is unerringly male. One wonders whether the progressive ejection of the feminine from the divinity does not reflect the progressive consolidation of the phenotype of maleness introduced in the first chapter. And one is left to wonder in which way the phenotype affected not only religion but science as well, including the very way of processing information and establishing what is important and what is not; and which gender is implicitly projected upon the very face of science.

The language of myth could be considered as a translation into mental images of collective, worldwide themes of adaptation and development as they are plausibly stored (as electrochemical patterns?) in the human brain. It is a robust language, shared by diverse cultures and phases of human development, which represents the creative expression of inner mental states in ways that are otherwise unequaled by modern, rationalistic thinking (where "unreasonable"

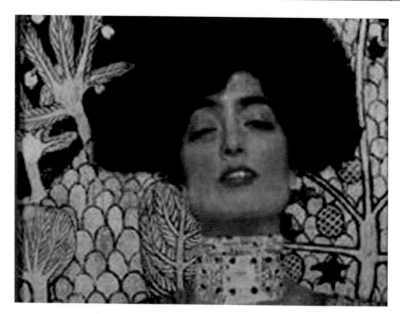

**Figure 3-1: Judith I, by G. Klimt, Osterreichische Galerie, Museum fur Ange-
wandte, Vienna, particular.** (Photo by author)

states have been by and large marginalized for the sake of rational purity).
It also represents the most enduring and international mode of thinking and
of communication, although its interpretation may be complex and ambiguous
and its vocabulary not exclusively verbal. The attributes of the eternal meanings
of the feminine as conceived by the patriarchies may have changed through
times and cultures, from the Paleolithic Venus through various goddesses of
old to the Judith of Klimt in Figure 3-1; but the mythical theme has persisted
and continues to thrive, in light as well as in darkness.

Recently, the mythical language has been shared by many scholars. Human-
ist Joseph Campbell (1973) describes how:

> The myths of man have flourished, and they have been the living inspiration of
> whatever else may have appeared out of the activities of the human body and mind.
> It would not be too much to say that myth is the secret opening through which
> the inexhaustible energies of the cosmos pour into human cultural manifestation.
> Religions, philosophies, arts, the social forms of primitive and historic man, prime
> discoveries in science and technology, the very dreams that blister sleep, boil up
> from the basic, magic ring of myth (p. 3).

Computer scientist David Gelernter explores in capturing detail the myth of
the Book of Exodus in order to illustrate the profound qualities of the language
of old, and comments: "the mind of these times ... let's say that it dates from
very roughly a thousand years BC—is quite capable of logic and reasoning

and ordinary, coherent narrative. But it remains comfortable, too, in cognitive neighborhoods where we no longer go, except in our dreams" (1994, p. 176).

Almost two millennia ago lecturer and philosopher Apuleius (1989) in his book The *Metamorphoses* reported in great detail the myth of Psyche (Figure 3-2). He probably constructed his narrative upon an older Greek version to which he may have added trimmings, as the Romans often did when adapting Greek themes to their own style. It is a complex, at times ambiguous and puzzling metaphor of the organization and unfolding of the human psyche. It possibly constitutes the most comprehensive and detailed extant version of the human mind written in the demotic language of the first-person perspective, from the point of view of the subjective experience.

The myth starts with a description of Psyche as the most beautiful and attractive virgin woman on Earth. She is so attractive that people flock to see her and the temples of Aphrodite stand deserted, which stirs the ire and jealousy of the goddess. If one looks at the opening drama more closely it becomes less clear why Aphrodite should be that jealous, given that no man actually wants Psyche, despite her beauty: "no prince or commoner wanted to marry her" (p. 245), but she is rather described as a perfectly polished statue, a "simulacrum fabre politum" and destined to remain forlorn and unwanted and to eventually be cast away. Actually, the Latin term *simulacrum* is more enigmatic than "statue"; it indicates something that represents something else, a simile, even a symbol. Still, Aphrodite is quite jealous of the young woman's attention. She calls her son Eros and commands him, with incestuous seductiveness, to go and kill Psyche. Eros promises to comply with her mother's wish.

In the meantime, Psyche and her parents come to the conclusion that all her beauty is a waste and indeed may bring sorrow to the town and shame to the family. By decree Psyche, dressed in her never-used nuptial robe, is accompanied to the top of a cliff and left there to die or to be the prey of some horrible monster (a not uncommon destiny in old times for young Greek daughters of displeased king-fathers).

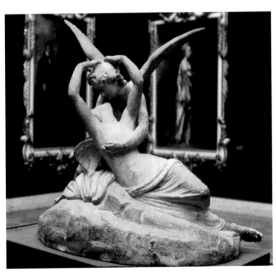

Figure 3-2: Amore e Psiche, by A. Canova, Musée du Louvre, Paris. (Photo by author)

When Eros arrives he finds Psyche sitting on the top of the cliff, weeping and lamenting; he is immediately pierced by one of his own arrows (not a few of those young Greek daughters escaped their fate by a last-minute divine intervention, as happened to Iphigenia as she was about to be executed by her father Agamemnon), falls in love with her, and asks the wind god Zephyrus to steal her away (the myth does not describe what lie he told mother).

Zephyrus complies: Psyche *falls asleep* and is carried by the wind to the bottom of the cliff. When she wakes up she sees in front of her a magnificent palace, the like of which she hasn't ever seen before. It appears to have been constructed not with human hands but by divine skills. In awe she walks inside and finds it to be immense, with an endless multitude of staterooms which, she realizes, contain "omnis mundi thesaurus"—the treasures of the entire world; "nec est quicquam quod ibi non est"—*nothing exists that is not there.*

An invisible servant, a voice without a body (corporis sui nuda) "comes to her" and addresses her stunned surprise by questioning why should she actually be surprised, given that all that lies around her is her own property; her exclusive property. As she can see there is no need for locks or doors or guards because no one else but Psyche could access the treasure.

This is an interesting angle to the story, given that the taking of such jealously guarded treasures as the Golden Fleece was often a glorious enterprise in those times; even the gods did not hesitate to steal precious items from each other if they thought they could get away with it. The invisible servants continue to anticipate every single one of Psyche's needs; they bathe her and feed her and entertain her. Eventually they bring her to her bed chamber and prepare her for the night. As is to be expected in a true love story, in the midst of the night she is joined by a male presence. He takes her and he tells her he will be her husband/lover forever (!) provided she agrees to receive him only under cover of darkness and to be satisfied with his commitment to her without trying to see his face. Should she see his face he will then have to leave her forever.[1]

Psyche is willing to go along with this and she begins to actually enjoy her husband. The myth describes how she cherished him, and gradually fell in love with the smell of cinnamon in his hair, the taste and texture of his skin, the way he touched her, and made love to her. While in this enhanced emotional state reached purely through "sensations" her creativity blossomed and she became pregnant. Her lover assured her that she was carrying a god-child.

At this point things got complicated. Competitiveness, sibling rivalry, jealousy, misinformation, and paranoia generated by the rest of Psyche's collective social system and sustained by the semblance of "rational" reasoning muddied

---

[1] Young lovers, divine or not, continue to not know the true meaning of "forever" and the transitory aspect of time.

the waters to the point where Psyche began to doubt the words of her lover and became convinced that she was carrying a monster and the son of a monster in her womb. Pressured by her sisters, one night she waited until her lover fell asleep; then she lit an oil lamp and approached the bed carrying a dagger, ready to plunge it into his heart. Predictably, as soon as the lamp lit Eros' face she fell completely and inexorably in love with him. At the same time a drop of the burning oil fell on his shoulder. Eros woke up and instantly disappeared! Psyche, dejected and desperate, started a long journey to find her true love. She went to the police, to administrators and bureaucrats, traveling all around the country (and it must have taken a long time, considering her pregnancy and the traveling conditions of that era), but all in vain. As is to be expected, all she got were vague suggestions or politically correct evasions. She even turned to the priests with even less success—Aphrodite was not a goddess to be taken lightly. Eventually, not knowing where else to turn, she went to prostrate herself at the feet of her not-so-nice putative mother-in-law and begged her to be allowed to see Eros.

The goddess was unrelenting. She told Psyche that she may as well go to hell first. This Psyche promptly did, in a very concrete way: she descended into Hell and met Persephone who felt pity for the young woman—and maybe secretly enjoyed creating a headache for her all-too-beautiful divine sister—and sent her unscathed back to Aphrodite carrying a vial of precious fragrance as a gift to the love goddess.

We are taught that curiosity kills the cat. On her way back Psyche figured that she had better use a little of the fragrance in order to become more attractive to Eros (and possibly to look a bit like his mother). She opened the vial and instantly fell into a deep, deathlike sleep.

Luckily for her, Zeus had by now grown tired of the entire melodrama. He called upon Aphrodite and pointed out to her how Eros himself had become seriously ill from the burning wound caused by Psyche and was close to death—a very embarrassing position for an Immortal to be in. An irritated Zeus was too much even for the goddess to handle and she "graciously" relented. She informed Eros of where to find Psyche. He immediately got better, flew to his beloved, raised her out of sleep, and both of them were this time integrated into the Pantheon as a properly married couple. There is no more mention of the pregnancy, which must have been well into the second trimester by the time Eros disappeared. The mother-to-be had then gone on the quest, by foot mostly, and waited endlessly for officials and their secretaries to do nothing. Persephone and Aphrodite did not mention the gestation, nor did Zeus. The myth, however, ends by saying, "and when the time came she gave birth to a daughter and her name was Pleasure" (p. 355).

I have presented the myth in a schematic fashion—the original version covers over 100 pages. This diagram of the mythical structure is sufficient for my present goal, to illustrate some major dimensions of the psychic phase space described in the demotic language: the polished and very attractive but ultimately sterile ego consciousness; the role of Eros in directing such consciousness toward creativity; the dimming of ego consciousness necessary for the transition to be actualized; the immensity and uniqueness of the content of data available to each psyche, as well as the surprise and incredulity that the ego experiences when faced with such treasure; the non-ego-conscious but highly rational decisional power of the self; the complex role that collective values may play in influencing the unfolding of the personal experience and of self-actualization. All myths seem to belong to their originators as well as to their interpreters, but in reality they belong to no one and to everyone. As I pointed out earlier on, "mythical reality becomes fundamentally a reality of humanity that involves universal concepts offering definition to particular ones. It is a structure gravid with timeless significance and always susceptible to recurrence" (see Chapter 1, p. 7). What I submit here is my interpretation of the myth of Psyche as I read it intersubjectively in the experience of Apuleius and with the support of past and present knowledge concurring with the material of the myth. Mind was of old perceived in this delightfully modern metaphor. It represents a piece of solid scientific research within its own rights.

Chapter 4

THE LANGUAGE OF THE OBJECTIVE OBSERVER: GERALD EDELMAN AND NEURODARWINISM: ANTONIO DAMASIO AND THE FEELING OF KNOWING

I mentioned in Chapter 1 how the suggestion that neurons in the human brain may act as functional groups reaches back at least to the beginning of the 20th century, when Sir Charles Sherrington offered the captivating metaphor of the enchanted loom. However, psychologist Donald Hebb (1949) was the first one to formulate the concept of the cell assembly in his classic book *The Organization of Behavior*. Hebb had been impressed by several phenomena that did not appear to fit with the assumptions of behaviorism.

The first set of conflicting data had to do with animal experiments, and specifically with his observation that chimpanzees (such as "Booie" and the other chimps he had worked with at Yerkes primate center) raised in a laboratory showed significant distress when presented with plaster casts of chimpanzee heads; these reactions, unrelated to previous experiences, seemed to indicate some fund of knowledge and deductive "reasoning" that did not fit behaviorally based expectations.

The second set of phenomena that attracted his attention had to do with the brain's resistance to traumas. An example of this was the famous case of Phineas Gage who had some part of his brain destroyed by a metal rod, over 3 feet long and almost 2 inches in diameter, which had shot through his skull, entering from the left cheek upward and exiting somewhere near the midline of the frontal vault. Mr. Gage had maintained most of his cognitive skills, despite the apparently massive destruction of frontal brain areas.[1] Hebb called this

---

[1] Most reports on the case, however, fail to illustrate the profound behavioral and affective changes that took place following the accident and practically destroyed Gage's life. A very illuminating study, complete with computerized reconstructions of the putative damage, can be found in Damasio (1994, pp. 3–33).

attitude of the nervous system *robustness*, referring to the fact that a damaged group of cells can recruit additional neurons to participate in its activities. Hebb proposed that nerve cells do not necessarily act as individuals in the dynamics of the brain, but rather as functional groups, which he called cell assemblies. He concluded that cells of an assembly might be widely dispersed over much of the brain (these assemblies were therefore conceptualized more as functional units than as anatomic ones) so that partial destruction of a brain area does not completely destroy any of the assemblies. He attributed to these assemblies of cells the following properties:

- Each complex assembly comprises a "three-dimensional fishnet" of many "thousands" of interconnected cells, sparsely distributed over much of the brain. The concept was a bold one, and it sat uncomfortably with the electroneurophysiologists of the late 1940s, who were already experiencing significant difficulties with single-neuron recordings. The idea of having to trace and consider the neuroelectrical field of "thousands" of cells was quite unpalatable and Hebb's theory was subjected to several decades of significant neglect.

- The interconnections among the cells of a particular assembly grow slowly in numbers and strength as a person matures, in response to both external stimuli and internal dynamics, tailored to the particular experiences of the organism. This was another significant insight that, in psychological terms, carries the following important messages: each human mind is a unique phenomenon; its structural organization is ever changing; what happens to a person plays an important and possibly fundamental role in how that person experiences the self and the world. The scientific inclination to support the primacy of the genetic message (today, "biological psychiatry" and the pharmaceutical industry strongly resonate in this direction, as I will comment in Chapter 11) found its balancing measure in this observation about the role of "nurture" and experience in the development of the human psyche—in health as well as in "illness."

- One mechanism suggested for the growth of neuronal interconnections postulates the strengthening of dendritic contacts through use. Hebb suggested that groups of neurons communicating with each other do not do so in a random way. Rather, the operation of communication is facilitated by the process of learning. Synaptic systems that interact with each other will continue to communicate in a preferential way, by developing stronger and easier links among themselves. Hebb coined the term *synaptic weighting* in order to define the phenomenon.

These Hebbian concepts have become the foundations of modern neuroscience (at least, of the one that I am familiar with): assemblies of neuronal networks (now viewed as comprising much greater numbers of cells than the "thousands" Hebb postulated) are the units of investigation for any unified theory; the lifelong process of dynamic adaptation is a given process; synaptic strengthening by preferred use is an operational standard.

Gerald Edelman and Neurodarwinism

Neuroscientist Gerald Edelman's theory of neuronal groups selection (TNGS; also known as neural Darwinism) (1988, 1989, 1992; Edelman &Tononi, 2000) offers a comprehensive example of a Hebbian model of neuronal functioning.[2] The latest elaboration of the model speculates about the translation of neural events into conscious mental images, although the hypothesis is as yet unproven.

The TNGS rests on three doctrines (Figure 4-1).

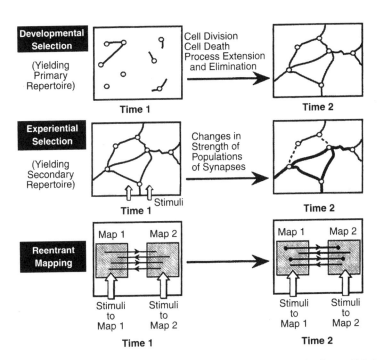

Figure 4-1: The theory of neuronal groups selection (TNGS, from Edelman & Tononi, 2000). (From: *A Universe of Consciousness: How Matter Becomes Imagination* by Gerald M. Edelman and Giulio Tononi. Reprinted by permission of Basic Books, a member of Perseus Books, L.L.C.)

---

[2] Another comprehensive "emergentist" neural model forms the subject of Scott's *Neuroscience* (2002).

1. The doctrine of *developmental selection* (DS) states that although the initial anatomy of the brain (that is, the formation of the neural plate and the neural groove or the migratory patterns of neural crest cells) rests on genetic information, from very early embryonic stages onward the *synaptic connectivity* of the neurons is guided by developmental selection. Anatomical synaptic links eventuate from topobiological competition (Edelman, 1988), involving, among other factors, cells being at specific places at specific times, and strengthened by joint firing of the neurons ("neurons that fire together wire together").

Those neurons that operate in synergy with each other are selected over those cells that remain dormant and eventually undergo cell death.[3] This selection in response to stimulus-response phenomena eventuates in sets of circuits that are highly diverse from one brain to the other.

2. *Experiential selection* (ES) states that "a lifelong process of synaptic selection occurs within each repertoire of neuronal groups as a result of experience" (Edelman & Tononi, 2000, p. 84). This process eventuates in *metastable synaptic organizations* that reflect the Hebbian law of synaptic weighting and favor certain pathways over others, although not at the level of single neurons—as described in the strict Hebbian formula—but acting upon whole populations of neurons.[4]

3. *Reentrant mapping*[5] is considered a central mechanism by Edelman. In his own words, *reentry* is described as "a process of temporally ongoing parallel signaling between separate maps along ordered anatomical connections" (Edelman, 1989, p. 49). It leads "to the synchronization of the activity of neuronal groups in different brain maps, binding them into circuits capable of temporally coherent output" (Edelman & Tononi, 2000, p. 85). "Brain maps are coordinated in space and time through ongoing signaling across reciprocal connections" (in the figure the dots in the maps represent strengthened synapses). Reentry requires a system of remarkable parallel connectivity to support its plasticity and its temporal coherence. Edelman and Tononi (2000) identify three major neuronal pathways (Figure 4-2).

1. *The thalamocortical system* (TGS) is formed by dense tracts of reentrant connectivity that connect the thalamic nuclei to specific areas of the cortex

---

[3] "Up to 70% of cells in a given area (of the nervous system) may die before the tissue is shaped" (Edelman, 1988, p. 13).

[4] Interestingly, when the synaptic network is stimulated by electrodes, the majority of synapses shows no detectable activity, these are called *silent synapses*. The silence, however, does not connote synaptic failure but rather selectional events occurring over the entire population of synapses in the region (Edelman, 1988, p. 207).

[5] For a detailed review of this fundamental process see Edelman (1989, pp. 64–90).

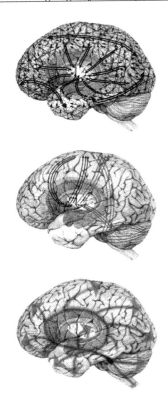

Figure 4-2: The three major connective systems (from Edelman & Tononi, 2000): TCS (top); PCS (middle); values systems (bottom). (From: *A Universe of Consciousness: How Matter Becomes Imagination* by Gerald M. Edelman and Giulio Tononi, Reprinted by permission of Basic Books, a member of Perseus Books, LX.C.)

and back. It includes also *corticocortical* fibers between different cortical areas (Edelman & Tononi, 2000).

2. *The parallel chains system* (PCS) is formed by long, polysynaptic loops arranged in parallel that leave the cortex, enter the *cortical appendages*, and return to the cortex.[6] The authors define as cortical appendages the *cerebellum* (supervises the coordination and synchrony of motion and plays a role in thought and language as well); the *basal ganglia* (involved in the planning and execution of complex motor and cognitive acts); and the *hippocampus* (plays a major role in consolidating short-term memory into long-term memory).

3. The noradrenergic, serotonergic, dopaminergic, cholinergic, and histaminergic *value systems* (VS) originate from relatively small areas and project in a diffuse manner all over the brain. These systems release neuromodulators in response to the occurrence of something important to the organism and influence neural activity as well as neural plasticity by determining changes in the strength of synaptic connections. Due to their diffusion throughout the brain these systems may in this way affect billions of synapses.

Incidentally, these changes in neural connectivity patterns over large areas could explain how assemblies of neurons may shift in their functional organization so that they may be involved in different functions linked with changes in their related value systems. If I understood correctly, this property includes what Edelman and Tononi (2000) refer to as degeneracy: "In (selected) systems there are typically many different ways, *not necessarily structurally identical*, by which a particular output occurs" (p. 86). Edelman and Tononi (2000) state:

> Sophisticated interactions among value systems related to pleasure, pain, bodily states, and various emotions are ... likely to govern cortical responses. The effects of value-dependent learning can range from the alignment of auditory and visual maps in the brain stem of the barn owl to the exquisite distinctions made by a connoisseur of wine or the emotional response of a guilty person. (p. 91)

The very categorization of reality itself is under the influence of these systems. At the moment we do not know how values are transmitted, nor do we know how "culture" affects the neural set of organizing values. If we briefly revisit the sexual value system that has been psychologically expounded by Freud we will probably come to agree with Mansfield (2000) in concluding that these sexual values have percolated upward out of the collective morals of a patriarchal society. They originate from a historical collective phenotype of predominance of maleness and become the "knowledge" upon which the brain will act; Freud's phallocentric articulation was actually not his "creation" but rather the reformulation in psychological terms of this predominant phenotype.

The task of identifying how value systems affect and balance each other, which loops, among these hierarchies of values, give eventually emergence to a specific individuality, and how they might be profoundly affected and changed within each subject by social and cultural influences, looks overwhelming. Occasionally, we get glimpses of such complexity and difficulty during therapeutic encounters, and, from a certain perspective, any successful resolution of a therapeutic process could be conceived as a rearrangement of values. I will return to these themes in Chapter 11.

As Figure 4-1 indicates, the final outcome of reentrant connectivity is the emergence of multiple *reentrant* local maps that can become dynamically integrated among each other and out of which dynamics a global structure could emerge: "A global mapping is ... a dynamic structure containing multiple reentrant local maps.... that interact with nonmapped regions, such as those of the brain stem, basal ganglia, hippocampus, and parts of the cerebellum" (Edelman & Tononi, 2000, p. 95). The reasoning suggesting that some brain areas may remain "nonmapped" is somewhat obscure, unless it is required in order to differentiate "consciousness-provoking" systems from those systems that may be considered insulated from the process of consciousness. This possible masked reason for Edelman and Tononi's articulation of their functional neuroanatomy will be readdressed in Chapters 5 and 6. Global maps evidently leave little neuroanatomy out of their organization and are considered precursors of the system postulated as necessary for the emergence of conscious mental phenomena. When activated, these global maps participate in a complex and temporally coherent system that allows for the emergence of consciousness: a *functional cluster*. In the words of Edelman and Tononi (2000):

A group of neurons can contribute directly to conscious experience only if it is part of a distributed functional cluster that, through reentrant interactions in the thalamocortical system, achieves high integration in hundreds of milliseconds .... We call such a cluster ... a "dynamic core" to emphasize both its integration and its constantly changing composition. (p. 144)

This brief review of the TNGS model outlines how brain processes can be formulated at several levels of description, from the dynamics of individual membrane proteins to the switching of isolated patches of membrane; up to the interaction among nerve impulses as they propagate along the neurons and modulate synaptic transmission and synaptic connectivity, to reach the intricate dynamics of repertoires of neurons, of assemblies of cells, and assemblies of assemblies that are coordinated first in local maps and then in global maps, and finally in neuronal clusters that extend over much of the brain.

Dr. Edelman's model is based on extensive observation of developmental and functional neuroanatomy as well as on computerized "virtual" models that explore connectivity itself and the processes that may influence it. The model offers a carefully elaborated, impressive example of "the observer's language" and is of great help in clarifying the "biological" arm, or dimension, of Psyche.

At present the TNGS model still falls short of filling the explanatory gap between electrochemistry and mental images, or "world knot," as Edelman and Tononi prefer to call it (2000, p. 3). The ongoing dilemma appears to be that "thought is a materially based process but is, itself, not material" (p. 157), a statement by Edelman and Tononi that closely recalls the position of William James that mind stuff is different from atom stuff, and underscores the complexity of having to face a biological domain simultaneously with a cognitive domain.

Antonio Damasio and the Feeling of Knowing

Edelman traces the neural buildup to the emergence of mental events and to consciousness, possibly in a way consistent with the implicit priority assigned to it by the philosophy of scientific materialism. He allocates a distinct place and importance to the "motus cordis" (if I am correct in considering his value systems as parts of affectivity; see Chapter 8) but his primary area of interest is the formation of neural representations that will eventuate in mental ones and in the progressive emergence of specific "types" of consciousness (see also Figure 5-1).

Neurologist and neuroscientist Antonio Damasio (1999) also has consciousness as his main subject, but he describes an operational system in which affectivity plays a major or even primary role (I will also retrace significant aspects of his work in the chapters on consciousness and affectivity).

Damasio approaches the biological basis of mind in a two-step sequence. In the first experimental step the behavior and the internal experiences of a subject, operating under predesigned conditions, are observed and measured. Consequently, the collected data are correlated to neurobiological information obtained from the simultaneous observation of known neurobiological systems (from molecules to systems of circuits). In his words: "The approach is based on the following assumptions: that the processes of the mind, including those of consciousness, are based on brain activity; that the brain is a part of a whole organism with which it interacts continuously; and that we, as human beings, in spite of remarkable individual traits that make each of us unique, share similar biological characteristics in terms of the structure, organization, and function of our organism" (p. 85).

Schematically, Damasio postulates a primary level of neural organization that he calls the neural self or *protoself*:

> *a coherent collection of neural patterns which map moment by moment the state of the physical structure of the organism in its many dimensions.* This ceaselessly maintained first-order collection of neural patterns occurs not in one brain place but in many, at a multiplicity of levels, from the brainstem to the cerebral cortex, in structures that are interconnected by neural pathways. (p. 154)

This neural pattern is evidently quite remote from a *mental pattern (or image)*.[7] The brain structures required for its implementation include several brainstem nuclei (responsible for the regulation of body states and body signals), the hypothalamus, which keeps track of several chemical and endocrine dimensions of the internal milieu, and the insular and somatosensory 2 cortices.

Interestingly, Damasio specifically excludes both hippocampus and cerebellum[8] from the neural systems supporting the neural maps of the protoself. As we have seen, these two structures are considered essential for map formation in the Edelman model, where they are an integral part of the parallel chain systems that represent one, and possibly the most essential, pathway required

---

[7] Damasio limits the term *neural pattern*, or map, to the neural aspect of the process (as the neural activities documentable by current neuroscientific methods "in activated sensory cortices").

[8] Damasio describes the hippocampus as "a vital structure in the on-line mapping of multiple concurrent stimuli" (p. 158) that receives information from, and reciprocates to, all sensory cortical areas via long polysynaptic parallel pathways (the parallel chain system of Edelman). It is also involved in the process of short-term memory and in the formation of permanent memories stored in other brain circuitries. Despite the role of the hippocampus in the formation of memories (that *have* to feed the architecture of images and the interaction of subject/object fundamental to core consciousness) Damasio states that "as far as consciousness goes," the role of the hippocampus is negligible (p. 333). He assigns to the cerebellum, "one of the most transparent but also elusive sectors of the brain" (p. 158), not only its traditional role in the modulation of fine movements, but also in emotions and in the search for specific verbal and nonverbal memories; its role in consciousness is described as "unclear" (p. 333).

for reentrant mapping. However, Damasio restricts the content of the first-order maps that form the neural self to first-order representations of current body states. He differentiates the dynamics that deal with this set of information from the dynamics that process the information concerning the "object," or what he also calls "something-to-be-known" (1999, p. 159),[9] The distinction is somewhat obscure to me for several reasons: first, at the neural levels implied here, any differentiating "knowledge" between stimuli does not admittedly exist[10] and, furthermore, the body could also be considered an "object," in many ways; second, in order to have core consciousness the protoself needs to be endlessly examined in the context of the subject-object relationship, which makes the distinction puzzling; finally, sensory input (either "internal" or "external") implies, inexorably, immediate (re) categorization, which implies involvement of previous experience that implies reflections on the protoself.

Beyond these two sets of neural structures—in which the causative object and the protoself are represented in a separate way—Damasio proposes "at least one other structure which re-represents[11] both protoself and object in their temporal relationship" (p. 177) and that constitutes a second-order neural pattern whose dynamics generate a second-order map. Among its main characteristics Damasio includes the ability to receive neural signals from the two dynamic structures assigned to the protoself and object representation, and the ability to "generate a neural pattern that 'describes,' in a temporally ordered manner, the events occurring in the first-order maps" (p. 177).

The superior culliculi, the cingulated cortex, the thalamus, and some pre-frontal cortices are listed among the brain structures putatively identified with this second-order neural pattern, as the sites "underlying the imaged account of the relationship and the enhancement of object image" (p. 191).

The *superior culliculi* are "multilayered structures which receive a multi-plicity of sensory inputs from an assortment of modalities, integrate signals in a complex fashion across these several layers, and communicate the resulting outputs to a variety of brainstem nuclei, the thalamus, and the cerebral cortex" (p. 264). They map the temporal and spatial attributes of the object as well as the characteristics of body state, and in this way affect cortical processing via reticular and thalamic nuclei and exert an effect on the cholinergic and monoaminergic value systems.

The *cingulated cortex* has a massive input from all divisions of the so-matosensory system describing the internal milieu as well as visceral and neuromuscular conditions. It is involved in a wide variety of motor activities in

---

[9] Parenthetically, he ultimately attributes the making of consciousness to the interaction between the brain maps of an organism and the brain maps of an "object."

[10] "The protoself has no power of perception and holds no knowledge" (p. 154).

[11] The model now runs parallel to Edelman's description of reentry and recategorization.

striatal and smooth muscles, and it is also involved in attention, emotion, and consciousness.

The *thalamus* "could signify the object-organism relationship in implicit form and follow that by creating more explicit neural patterns in cingulated cortices and somatosensory cortices" (p. 265).

Finally, a sustained and expanded state of core consciousness forms the foundation for *extended consciousness* (see Chapter 5 for further discussion of extended consciousness and the related concept of the autobiographical self). This condition represents the ongoing activation of the processes described above; "the capacity to be aware of a large compass of entities and events ... over a larger compass of knowledge than that surveyed in core consciousness" (1999, p. 198). Damasio appears to identify this functional brain state with what he calls "the autobiographical self." As its anatomical basis he postulates an *image space* in which are contained all the images that have actually happened, and *a dispositional space* that contains the knowledge out of which images could be constructed.[12] He defines dispositions as "abstract records of potentialities." Higher-order cortices hold dispositions, or records of knowledge. They are held in neuronal ensembles that Damasio calls *convergence zones* (Damasio, 1999, pp. 219, 333). "To the partition of cognition between an image space and a dispositional space, then, corresponds a partition of the brain into (1) neural-pattern maps, activated in the early sensory cortices, the so-called limbic cortices, and some subcortical nuclei, and (2) convergence zones, located in the higher-order cortices and in some subcortical nuclei" (pp. 219–220).

I have already mentioned how the foundation for Edelman's model is formed by an extensive analysis of the processes of natural selection (genetic constraints, developmental selection, experiential selection) that confront the development of neurons and dictate their structural and functional organization. This organization is explored through virtual robotic models built to mirror progressive levels of increasing brain complexity.

In Damasio's model the dynamics of the structural and functional (micro) cytoarchitecture of the brain are given no apparent attention; his "pointers of the anatomy of the nervous system" (p. 324) deal practically with the macroanatomy of the brain. The model rests on laboratory data from experimental human subjects, and primarily from observations of neuropathology.[13] Clinical cases are analyzed and interpreted in order to offer insight and support to the theoretical model. Epileptic automatism, akinetic mutism (or locked-in

---

[12] We find here a strong echo of the phase space describing the *dimension of creativity* mentioned on p. 24.

[13] Damasio (1999) notes: "The investigation of patients with neurological disease has shaped my view on consciousness more than any other source of evidence" (p. 86).

syndrome) and Alzheimer's are seen as disturbances in core consciousness that confirm it "through its absence" (p. 94); transient global amnesia, anosognosia (or hemineglect) and asomatognosia (or temporary loss of one's own body perception) are seen as disturbances in extended consciousness and in the autobiographical self.[14]

To conclude this first part and the presentation of the three languages, I suggest a general guiding rule: the formulation and application of the third-person and first-person languages to the study of mind, and in my opinion to the clinical arena as well, need to reflect, and be consistent with, the ideographic language of the set of rules that define all biological phenomena. Whenever the "translation" becomes muddled or forced, then probably something is "fishy" concerning the psychological or the biological metaphors.

---

[14] The issue of the relationship between neuropsychophysiology and neuropsychopathology will be revisited at several points in later chapters.

PART II

Seeking the Understanding

Chapter 5

CONSCIOUSNESS

In Chapter 1, I traced how, during the last few centuries, Western thought and Western science came to articulate the phenomenon, or state of mind, of consciousness. As a consequence of an enhanced preoccupation for "rational" consciousness, the awareness and curiosity for the nonconscious dimensions of mind gradually faded away in the West, the process being accelerated by the discomfort with elusive aspects of the topic that has plagued the materialistic philosophy of science.[1]

The uneasiness concerning subjectivity is perhaps well illustrated by a web search that I conducted in April 2002 at the Barnes and Noble site. I found over 5,000 books that carried the word consciousness in their titles. A random check indicated that at least 70% of these books dealt with the argument from a neuropsychological perspective, as a topic of study or research. By comparison, the word subjectivity appeared in the title of approximately 400 books. These were reviewed in as much detail as the information available at the site allowed. Only a handful dealt with the topic from a neuropsychological perspective. The majority reflected either an aesthetic or a sociopolitical or a philosophical perspective.

What is consciousness? I submit a few among the many definitions available:

1. "The moment we try to fix our attention upon consciousness and to see what, distinctly, it is, it seems to vanish" (G. E. Moore, 1903, p. 450, as reported by William James [cited in Wilshire, 1984, p. 164]).

---

[1] Philosopher John Searle (1992) pointed out that the reason for the fear that consciousness has triggered in scientists is that "consciousness has the essentially terrifying feature of subjectivity" (p. 55). Consciousness has therefore to be disconnected from the subjective component, and transformed into a quantifiable or a marginal feature of mind.

2. "Consciousness connotes a kind of *external relation*, and does not denote a special stuff or way of being" (W. James cited by Wilshire, 1984, p. 172; emphasis added).[2]
3. "A sense-organ for the perception of psychic qualities" (S. Freud).
4. "A fascinating but elusive phenomenon: it is impossible to specify what it is, what it does, or why it evolved. Nothing worth reading has been written about it" (International Dictionary of Psychology, 1989).
5. "A unified mental pattern that brings together the object and the self" (Damasio, 1999, p. 11).

All well and good, but not terribly illuminating. Let us see what happens if we try to probe into the phenomenon in a different way, by correlating the analyzable information available through the three languages. Such correlation should emphasize and validate common characteristics and attributes, and allow us to reframe them in a multidimensional view. It could also outline differences and permit their evaluation from more than one perspective.[3]

In the language of nonlinear dynamics, consciousness is considered as an emergent phenomenon from the dynamics of complex systems of neural assemblies and the interaction with the higher levels of the cognitive hierarchy, as the level of culture. As Scott states in introducing the phenomenon, "it should be no surprise that consciousness, a biological reality even to children, is yet another instance of such nonlinear coherence. Consciousness *emerges...*" (Scott, 1995, p. 5). Therefore, while all the repeated experimentation on consciousness in subsets of human subjects allows the formulation of rules that pose constraints and specify a framework (for instance, it needs a brain: a computer won't do; it needs a lot of brain, a Petri dish of neurons won't suffice; specific brain regions may be required, but no region is per se sufficient; and so on), its emergence appears also linked to the dynamics of permutable factors, none of which could be a priori excluded because they all participate to the functional and global organization of the cognitive hierarchy. In other words, while a certain level of involvement of the neural substrate is necessary for its emergence, one cannot predetermine which factors—or levels in the hierarchy—might be consistently and predictably included or excluded; indeed, the recursive causal loops imply immense flexibility and happenstance, and the phase space requires that all possible coordinates be considered—at least

---

[2] James also states that the word stands not for an entity but for a function (Wilshire, 1984, p. 163). In the second chapter of Principles of Psychology he asks: "But is the consciousness which accompanies the activity of the cortex the only consciousness that man has? Or are his lower centers conscious as well?"

[3] The constant theme to be kept in the forefront is that all metaphors carry the validity of the minds behind them, provided their "creation" represents the outcome of serious programmatic search on the matter in question.

potentially—in the eventuation of the process.[4] This is an important frame of reference: all models require sufficient compliance with it, in order to be considered as viable candidates.

What has the objective language of neuroscience to say concerning consciousness? This language conforms basically to the same position postulated by nonlinear physics, as exemplified in the phrase by Edelman and Tononi (2000) "We emphatically do not identify consciousness in its full range as arising solely in the brain, since we believe that higher brain functions require interaction both with the world and with other persons" (p. 199).

Both neuroscientific models presented in Chapter 4 tend to subdivide the phenomenon in modules distributed along a dimension of increasing complexity. Edelman and Tononi postulate two forms of consciousness:

1. *Primary consciousness*, or the ability to generate a mental scene in which a large amount of information is integrated for the purpose of directing present or immediate behavior.
2. *Higher-order consciousness* (HOC), or primary consciousness plus a sense of self and the ability in the waking state explicitly to construct and connect past and future scenes.

In the previous chapter I have outlined the progression of neural organization that Edelman and Tononi consider to be the requirement for the emergence of consciousness. Figure 5-1 schematically illustrates the steps and mechanisms involved in the emergence of primary consciousness and of the higher-order type (what Edelman calls "conscious of being conscious").

It is interesting to note the difference in the content and in the presumed organization of the two "bootstraps" involved in the process of eliciting consciousness. The *perceptual bootstrap* could be plausibly organized as primary electrochemical processes that translate into the "dialect" of neurons the sensory information provided by the interaction of the organism with itself and with the environment. The information is far richer and the dialect infinitely more complex than their aneuronal protozoan equivalents; but the

---

[4] At the level of the nerve membrane, consciousness can be altered by chemicals that bind to membrane proteins and block ionic transport across the membrane. At the level of the neuron, consciousness is routinely switched off and on by anesthetic agents that change the action of the synaptic contacts between cells. At higher levels, one is conscious of something called thought, which is stored in myriad complex assemblies that have been pieced together throughout the years of learning. Thought, in turn, is formed by and interacts with the culture in which it develops. Up and down the hierarchy, from membrane ion channels to the ebb and flow of cultural interactions, an intense intercourse between the levels continues (Scott, 1995, p. 172).

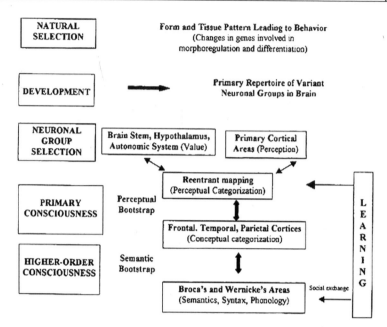

Figure 5-1: "The evolution of consciousness depends on the evolution of new morphology. Here, an evolutionary sequence of events is shown in which the principles of natural selection and development lead to neural recognition systems and result in conscious experience. No new principles besides those of the theory of neuronal group selection are required.... Notice that a 'perceptual bootstrap' produces primary consciousness and a 'semantic bootstrap' produces higher-order consciousness. Both bootstraps rely on the evolution of appropriate reentrant pathways in the brain." (Adapted from *Bright Air, Brilliant Fire* by Gerald M. Edelman, 1992, p. 134, with the permission of the author, Basic Books Inc. [Copyright © 1998].) Reprinted by permission of Basic Books, a member of Perseus Books. L.L.C.

basic mechanism may be seen as comparable. This complex machinery can be easily visualized as operating fully out of the realm of consciousness.[5]

The *semantic bootstrap*, however, in my opinion presupposes the *formation of mental images*. Its fundamental source of information is learning, which presumes the gradual understanding of abstract symbols, semantic or otherwise. In fact, the type of stimuli implied by Edelman (to which one could add ethical and religious value systems, integers, and other mathematical "universals," the appreciation of the difference between the language of poetry and that of prose, and so on) do not operate via the sensory system as much as they

---

[5] We may have differences of opinion about which type of consciousness is involved in these processes.

do via consciousness itself, self-reflective learning being a good example of my point. The entire world of abstract learning is a world of mental images. Higher-order consciousness requires that incredibly complex positive loops— or reentrant mappings—operate at the other side of the explanatory gap, within the category of mental images.[6]

Damasio submits a similar subdivision of consciousness into two modules of which the first is a prerequisite for the second. However, his model is complicated by the identification of these states of consciousness with specific forms of selfhood. He regards "the problem of consciousness as the combinations of two intimately related problems" (p. 9). Schematically, he states that consciousness requires the capacity for the brain to form mental images (descriptive, affective, dynamic) of the "object" and "of the self in the act of knowing" (p. 9); and also requires the interaction between these two sets of mental representations. He subdivides the outcome of this interaction in two different states that reflect a different temporal attribute:

1. *Core CSN:* A simple, biological phenomenon that provides the biological organism with a sense of self about the here and now.
2. *Extended CSN:* Coming with many levels and grades, it provides an elaborate sense of self: an identity as a person.

However, as we encountered during my brief review of Damasio's model, things are actually complicated by an earlier state that he calls protoself (to be consistent, should it be also called protoconsciousness?). Damasio's central focus on the concept of selfhood is underscored by how his entire narrative is based on the use of these terms and the exploration of these self-structures, under such headings as "The making of Core Consciousness" (p. 168) or "Extended Consciousness" (p. 198). Table 5-1 summarizes these different self-organizations that in part reflect also different types of consciousness.

Damasio's autobiographical self (and extended consciousness) appears to be congruent with the HOC of Edelman and Tononi; his core self (and core consciousness) appear congruent with their primary consciousness concept.

Damasio's model is also consistent with Edelman and Tononi's model in that once consciousness is achieved mental images exist as "such" *and* as electrochemical events, the two states endlessly reproposing themselves as two different representations of the same structures, responding to different demands or functions that at the moment keep evading us.[7]

---

[6] Incidentally, I am of the opinion that these mental images coexist as electrochemical organizations, "shifting" between two modes of presentation depending upon unknown factors (the requirement to communicate internally as well as externally could be one factor) and via unknown mechanisms. If this is correct then the feedback loops operate across the gap itself.

[7] As I mentioned previously in discussing this point in Edelman's model, I have come to the conclusion that the "mental" translation has an interactive function. In a previous book

Table 5-1: Kinds of self (modified from Damasio, 1999, pp. 174, 175).

Autobiographical Self
Based on permanent but dispositional records of core-self experiences. These records can be activated as neural patterns and turned into explicit images, and are partly modifiable with further experience. They constitute an autobiographical memory that contains memories of past experiences and of the anticipated future. We are conscious of the autobiographical self.

Core Self
Represents the second-order nonverbal account that occurs whenever an object modifies the protoself. The core self can be triggered by any object. The mechanism of production of core self undergoes minimal changes across a lifetime. We are conscious of the core self.

Consciousness

Protoself
An interconnected and temporally coherent collection of neural patterns which represent the state of the organism, moment by moment, at multiple levels of the brain. We are not conscious of the protoself.

These systems present us with very valuable insights into the neural mechanisms underlying consciousness and are thought provoking. If some areas trigger critical comments, and they do, probably these are due more to limitations in the language and lack of adequate mental metaphors than to anything else. Two such areas, having to do with the "classification" itself, attracted my attention.

1. Core CSN and primary CSN are presented as well-known and well-identified phenomena. Actually, it seems that most of the "real" evidence in support of core consciousness and primary consciousness stems from neuropathology. I am not aware of any objective confirmation of this type of consciousness in healthy humans, under physiological conditions. As I mentioned earlier on, Damasio constructs this state from the observation of patients with absence seizure and automatisms (1999, p. 86). I am skeptical at the implication that pathological consciousness belongs to the same class as physiological consciousness, given our ignorance concerning the neurodynamics of consciousness. It would indeed be difficult to "isolate," under physiological rather than pathological conditions, the hypothetical core type from more time-extended manifestations of consciousness.

2. There is also a reductionistic flavor to the way the process is described. Both systems seem to imply that extended consciousness represents the buildup

---

(Sanguineti, 1999, pp. 35–34) I exposed in detail—although from an essentially psychological, first-person perspective—my inferences about these two different types of thought organization, which I labeled "very rapid thinking" (VRT) and "relational thinking" (RT).

of repeated recurrences of the simpler type—Damasio actually considers the extended form as the result of "continuous pulses of core consciousness" accompanied by continuous reactivations of the autobiographical memory system (p. 199). This facade of reductionism—attempts to break down consciousness into smaller modules and then reconstruct it through a linear assembly—may just be only a facade. However, when Damasio states that "the mechanism of production of core self undergoes minimal changes across a lifetime" (p. 174) he seems to suggest that the functional workings out of which core consciousness emerges are not susceptible to positive feedback; in other words, they are not part of dynamic loops with higher hierarchical levels, nor are they subjected to downward, formal causative influences.

We have seen that such a unidirectional, linear type of function is not compatible with the biological organism because it could not deal with the complexity and the multidimensionality already present at this level of the hierarchy. It could indeed help to revisit some of the dimensions involved and listed by Damasio: "In short: As the brain forms images of an object— such as a face, a melody, a toothache, the memory of an event—and as the images of the object *affect* the state of the organism, yet another level of brain structures creates a swift nonverbal account of the events that are taking place in the varied brain regions activated as a consequence of the object-organism interaction. The mapping of the object-related consequences occurs in first-order neural maps representing protoself and object; the account of the *causal relationship* between object and organism can only be captured in second-order neural maps" (p. 170).

If one adds to the dimensions implied in this interaction those related to the protoself ("the key aspects... provided in the proto-self [are]: the state of internal milieu, viscera, vestibular system, and musculoskeletal frame" [p. 170]) it becomes evident that any reductionistic approach would be faced with the scale and complexity of difficulties outlined in Chapter 2, and that the causal relationships mentioned above have to reflect self-sustaining loops and bidirectionality among events.[8]

This analysis illustrates the usefulness of reframing mental events in more than one language: in this case, the application of the appropriate language of

---

[8] Evidence for such bidirectionality could be accrued by the same method used by Damasio: the field of medical pathology is rich with examples of short-or long-term downward causation exercised upon the fields of the protoself by higher-level events. The jet-lag phenomenon could be an instance of the impact of external, environmental changes upon the mechanisms of the protoself. The moving out of the time zone to which internal clocks are adjusted (as well as the moving back into the zone) triggers the emergence of a syndrome that illustrates the resistance as well as the degree of adaptive flexibility; I have not investigated the issue but I suspect that sleep is not the only function to be modified; probably other inner clocks, as the hormonal pulses, also become affected and formally readjusted to reflect the changes in higher-level dynamics.

universal rules, within which all biological phenomena need to be enclosed in order to maintain substance, clarifies what could otherwise be a significant misunderstanding in the process of consciousness.

I have another, more personal and philosophical reservation about the consciousness hierarchy, however. The definition also implies that man is substantially different from the rest of creation: man is the only biological organism entitled to higher-order consciousness. How much time each species spends in being conscious before having to start being conscious all over again is to me a mystery, and the entire species-demarcated approach may only reflect the emotional investment of humanity to differentiate itself psychologically in a categorical way from all other biological organisms.[9]

To summarize: The objective language describes consciousness as the outcome of a progression in neural dynamics that eventually involve most if not all of the brain and finds further expansion along the dimension of time. The progressive organizing process of neural events described in these two models (with its greatest emphasis in the TNGS one) finds a very fitting correlation in the system of hierarchies postulated by nonlinear science and adheres harmoniously with the dynamics expounded by that set of physics. The "flat" dimension of neuronal distribution and activation described in the language of the objective observer assumes depth when it becomes conceptualized also in terms of the universal rules that regulate life: neural events become dynamic loops of bidirectional causation and eventually contribute to phase spaces that signify "single" entities in which the energies of innumerable "components" are reorganized into a single emergent outcome "greater than the sum of its parts."

What could the first-person language of psychology contribute to the theme of consciousness and to the related theme of the self? Some psychological sciences have repeatedly suggested a different subdivision in ego consciousness and self-consciousness (or ego and self). This subdivision does not imply any reductionism: self-consciousness is not the product of the sum of many ego states. These two organizations represent different functions—or, perhaps more accurately, the ego represents a specific function of the self (many aspects of the self are not accessible or visible to the ego). These organizations are familiar and intersubjectively accessible to the psychological scientist, while the neuroscientist may not be as conversant with their characteristics, due to the different language used and to the reliance on the Cartesian concept of consciousness.[10]

---

[9] A categorical difference eliminates the discomfort that we would experience if we had to admit that we might be eating cognizant minds.

[10] At the cost of being redundant I want to stress again that from the psychological perspective equating, and therefore limiting, mind to (Cartesian) higher-order consciousness (Edelman & Tononi, 2000, p. 190) is in my opinion another serious categorical error.

The psychological states of the ego and of the self imply two different perspectives, two different points of view, when attempting to approach the function of consciousness: the point of view of the self or that of the ego. Paraphrasing Jung (1958, p. 15), anyone who has ego consciousness takes self-knowledge for granted; but, as I mentioned earlier, the ego knows only its own content; it does not know the unconscious component of the self and its content.

Naturally, the suggestion that a decisional structure may organize and direct the subject outside of ego awareness can represent a serious threat to the perception of one's identity when the culture (inclusive of science) to which the individual belongs supports an exclusively Cartesian type of selfhood. We have seen, however (Chapter 1), how the ego/self model has been an intuitive presence and a constant source of puzzled acknowledgment that generated multiple "explanations" throughout history. In the myth of Psyche the heroine stands for the ego, the rational mind; the unseen "servants" (invisible consciousness) realize her needs, and their decisional processes eventuate in "voices" directing ego consciousness (the profound role of Eros will be visited in Chapter 8).

If one substitutes self in place of brain, this description correlates closely with Damasio's statement *"The brain knows more than the conscious mind reveals"* (1999, p. 42) and the two functions could be schematized as in Table 5-2.

Differently put, is consciousness limited to *outcomes* of thought or does it involve also the *process* of thinking?[11] Along this line of reasoning, a related issue is whether consciousness is indeed the either-or phenomenon that is implied in Edelman and Tononi's model (either the dynamic core is activated, once events reach a critical mass, or is not), a condition that leaves no space for such ambiguous states as dreams, or the fringe phenomena described by William James, or even the dissociative states that are discussed by Damasio.

If we expand on the well-accepted and shared view that consciousness is a function of the brain that emerged out of some evolutionary need—an invaluable and fundamental function[12]—we could then begin to ask ourselves how this event would best fit the general organization of biological organisms.

---

[11] This is a very interesting and complex question. Edelman and Tononi (2000) pose the question and present their own answer: "Is thought necessarily always conscious? Whatever the play between the conscious and the unconscious and however strongly unconscious *routines* may, at times, overwhelm conscious decisions, thought itself, in our view, requires consciousness" (p. 206; emphasis added). I will critically revisit this conclusion, and the entire issue, in the next chapter.

[12] Damasio is of the idea that consciousness prevailed in evolution because knowing the feelings caused by emotions was indispensable for the art of life. He states: "consciousness was invented so that we could know life" (1999, p. 31).

Table 5-2: Ego and self-consciousness.

Consciousness of the Ego	Consciousness of the Self
The state we are in now	Largely nonconscious to the ego
"Higher-order consciousness" or	Binding and ongoing
conscious of being conscious	Not only relational
Relational?	Complete awareness
Binding quality	Atemporal?
Very limited awareness	

Schematically, if the brain is an organ of the body[13] and if consciousness is a function of the brain, then the brain and consciousness operate as all other organs and functions of the body: they do not ever stop. They simply undergo changes in their level of activity.

If this formulation is acceptable and consistent with what we know about biology, then:

1. Ego consciousness is just *one* manifestation of this complex cerebral function. Ego consciousness is fundamental in providing the brain with new information that is needed when the subject is faced with new "tasks" to be processed in order to navigate the environment (particularly when these tasks require multiple choices).[14] It may primarily represent an interactive function of the self, the way that the brain uses to communicate to others and to exist within the social network.
2. The level of self-consciousness reflects both internal and external requirements. In sleep the ego may be partially or fully unconscious but the self maintains a variable level of consciousness, as manifested by dreams and various levels of awareness of the environment as well as of plans for action (consider the need for an early awakening due to a planned trip).
3. This complex and continuous processing of the internal and external environment constitutes our subjective world, the content of the palace of Psyche.

---

[13] One could be justified in considering the evolution of the brain and its "higher" functions not only from the advantage of a "central station" for all information, but primarily as essentially an organ of choice and elaboration of alternatives, which gradually complemented, and improved upon, the strict genetic intelligence that offered stability of tested patterns but inferior ability to deal with adaptive changes. This process gradually evolved complex patterns of adaptation with only moderate penetrance but malleable to variations that reflect the needs of the species and of the individual.

[14] A simple but telling example is driving: in this activity we can routinely observe the difference between automatic behavior (the unconscious routines and subroutines described by Edelman and presented in the next chapter) when we reenact a known path, and the immediate activation of the ego whenever we have to select a "lateral" choice or to discover a completely new route.

My emphasis on the reevaluation of the meaning of consciousness is not solely based on semantics. The matter has very profound implications and I will discuss some of them in part III of the book. In my opinion, neuroscience in general has brought outstanding contributions to the workings of the brain. The actual contribution to the understanding of consciousness constitutes a very different matter; it is still quite tentative at best, despite the fact that a significant amount of neuroscientific work has been described under the label of "consciousness research." Mental images continue to slip away from neural patterns because of their different languages: the latter are also traceable electrochemical phenomena, while the former are as yet exclusively personal utterances. Therefore neuroscience will become a science of consciousness only by incorporating the two languages and by revising its conceptualization of the stream of consciousness.

Chapter 6

THE UNCONSCIOUS

The relationship between the conscious and the unconscious aspects of mind is evidently a fundamental one but, as already described in Chapter 1, it has been riddled with obstacles and fundamental problems since its inception. It is a fascinating topic, and nowhere is the split better exemplified than at the level of the scientific community: consider the weight on consciousness that pervades neuroscience in comparison with the weight on the unconscious permeating a substantial part of the psychological sciences.

I will use as a base two statements that sound reasonable and generally applicable:

1. If the visible part of mind deserves all the consideration that I outlined in the previous chapter, then the invisible part should require at least the same attention.
2. If we find that the information about consciousness is complex and often ambiguous, the information about the unconscious is only much more so, given—among other sources of difficulty—the fact that it is by definition described as unconscious and invisible. An analysis of the second statement is crucial, because, as will become evident during the following discussion, it mirrors the common refrain in justifying why the study of the unconscious aspects of mind has to be avoided out of necessity, in order not to muddle scientific research.

That being said, let us look again, as we did in the case of consciousness, to what the information written in the three languages has to say about the unconscious and its relationship with the conscious experience.

Nonlinear science is overall silent on the topic.[1] The reason may reside in the fact that, while conscious awareness and conscious thoughts are visible

---

[1] When I recently questioned this silence with Scott, he reminded me how D. Hebb makes some points that are related to the unconscious mind. Considering subliminal perception, in

phenomena, they are nevertheless intrinsically entwined with the dynamics out of which they emerge. As a storm, or a poem, or the flame of a candle, consciousness is an expression of multiple self-sustaining systems, none of which could be considered in isolation from the others. A similar perspective can be construed concerning the unconscious dynamics of mind; they too emerge continuously out of the complex interactions along the levels of the hierarchy. We need to remind ourselves that some of these levels are subject to empirical verification, while others are not; these last speculative levels include:

Complex assembly
Assembly of assemblies of assemblies
Assembly of assemblies
Assembly of neurons

These are presumably the levels where the world knot is tied—or the explanatory gap filled—the levels where the unconscious workings of the brain assume increasing substance and meaningful organization, and neurochemical patterns become mental ones.[2]

The unified field of dynamics from which consciousness emerges offers a strong basis for the versatility and adaptive capability that possibly represented the major evolutionary requirements dictating the (progressive) development of the human mind. That all information stored in the brain be always and completely potentially available to any and all adaptive situations is an incredibly difficult concept to digest; but so is the connectivity of the human brain.

Neuroscience appears to have a lot to say about unconscious dynamics and the role that such unconscious structures play in the overt content of mind. What it actually says is another matter. Edelman and Tononi (2000) introduce their position concerning the unconscious by affirming that "unconscious aspects of mental activity, such as motor and cognitive routines, and so-called unconscious memories, intentions, and expectations play a fundamental role in shaping and directing our conscious experience." They maintain that: "The dynamics of the core can be powerfully affected by a set of neural routines that are triggered by different core states and that, once completed, help bring about yet other core states." And continue: "We also discuss the possibility that islands of activity in the thalamocortical system may coexist with the core, influence its behavior, and yet not be incorporated in it" (p. 170). They proceed

---

Hebb's view, latent assemblies are partially stimulated, but not to the level of consciousness. This leaves them with lowered thresholds for stimulation into full firing—or consciousness.

[2] Are there actual indications for the existence of this "dynamic unconscious" apart from the speculations of theoretical psychology? I will address this profound question, in my own way, after some further review of the information available through the other languages.

to describe different functional modules of unconscious activity for which they propose specific neurophysiological frameworks.

1. One set represents neural activities similar to the circuitry that regulates blood pressure. These neural activities "not only remain unconscious but are completely inaccessible to the core and therefore to conscious monitoring and control" (p. 171). However, they can be responsive to "feedback" (p. 171).[3]

2. While reasserting the constant reciprocal influence between the conscious experience and unconscious processes (p. 177)[4] they describe a second set of neural activities that comprises all automatic routines and subroutines as "the player's fingers (operating) without conscious control until the player gives some conscious directive ... during the execution of the piece" (p. 177).[5] Edelman and Tononi propose that these "automatic routines and subroutines that interface with the core" are probably implemented by a series of polysynaptic loops that leave the thalamocortical system (p. 183) and subsequently make their way back there.

3. On the other hand, these authors:

> In order not to indulge in speculative neurology... resist the temptation to suggest possible neural mechanisms for aspects of unconscious cognition that, while having obvious psychological significance, are *far removed from neurophysiological understanding*. We refer, for instance, to the role of unconscious contexts, such as unconscious expectations and intentions, in shaping conscious experience—to the conscious and unconscious regulation of attention; and to the substrates and mechanisms of the Freudian unconscious. (p. 178; emphasis added)

This statement points to the complexity inherent to the study of "invisible" phenomena and from this viewpoint the caution exercised in addressing this last set of modules of unconscious activity appears sound, until one considers that the dynamic core is also a highly speculative neurological metaphor (Figure 6-1).

There is a puzzling and even subtly dismissive message in this insistence on a separation between the emergence of consciousness and unconscious dynamics, and in the implicit rejection of the idea that the neural mind—or

---

[3] The phenomena of "white coat hypertension" (increase in blood pressure when faced with a physician in an examining room) and its substantial response to conscious relaxation question such complete insulation between conscious experience and these neural patterns.

[4] "Conscious experience does not just float freely above an ocean of functionally insulated, unconscious processes. Instead, it is constantly influencing and being influenced by many unconscious processes ... conscious and unconscious processes are regularly in touch and their separation is often far from clear."

[5] Whoever saw pianist Keith Jarrett playing, for example, witnessed an immensely more complicated set of "unconscious" motoric activity involving the entire body that would better fit a definition of creative thoughts than the definition of being a routine or subroutine.

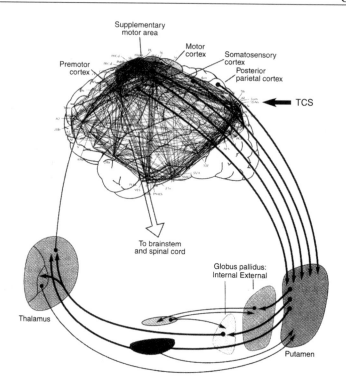

Figure 6-1: Structures and connections mediating conscious and unconscious processes. The TCS arrow (added by the present author) points to the thalamo-cortical system, "represented by a fine meshwork of cortical and thalamic areas and reentrant connections." This system is the neurophysiological representation of the functional cluster and dynamic core. The figure also depicts the parallel fibers systems to one appendage (basal ganglia) and back to the thalamus (here represented "outside" but actually intrinsically part of the meshwork) (Edelman & Tononi, 2000, p. 174). (From: *A Universe of Consciousness: How Matter Becomes Imagination* by Gerald M. Edelman and Giulio Tononi. Reprinted by permission of Basic Books, a member of Perseus Books, L.L.C.)

phase space or dynamic core—could be the neurophysiological substrate for the unconscious as well as for consciousness.[6]

4. Indeed, Edelman and Tononi conclude by proposing another set of unconscious processes. "One last category of unconscious neural processes may occur ... in the thalamo-cortical system that ordinarily participate in

---

[6] In other words, it baffles me why would this field of mental dynamics be more removed from neurophysiological understanding than the field of dynamics that eventuate in consciousness. I would (and will) push the identification forward and state that the dynamic core is the dynamic unconscious and consciousness (HOC) simply reflects an emergent threshold event within such unconscious system.

the core but that, under certain conditions, may remain functionally insulated from it" (Edelman & Tononi, 2000, p. 189). They notice that: "The possibility that splinter cores or autonomously functioning thalamo-cortical breakaways may exist alongside a dominant core raises several intriguing questions" (p. 190). So, Edelman and Tononi finally formulate the neural dynamics of the dynamic unconscious, but as splintered aspects of conscious dynamics. This is consistent with their being centered on their conceptualization of consciousness (specifically HOC, or conscious of being conscious).

This separation between the dynamics participating in consciousness and different types of unconscious dynamics does not seem to fit the nonlinear model of recursive events among assemblies and assemblies of assemblies and so on, to which Edelman and Tononi's reentry processes, their local and global maps, and the dynamics among the elements of the distributed functional clusters, carry an otherwise impressively close correlation.[7]

Damasio's position about unconscious activities sounds different in a substantial way from the position of Edelman and Tononi. The difference possibly reflects: (1) the different role of emotions in the two models; (2) the fact that Damasio's extended consciousness—and the underlying autobiographical self-paradigm—has some similarity to the self-consciousness model I submitted in the preceding chapter; (3) his continuous focus on the brain as a site of organized knowledge while Edelman seems to focus on consciousness as the site of knowledge;[8] (4) maybe even diversity in ethnic and cultural templates operative within the scientists' minds (see Chapter 7).

Damasio (1999) traces an "unconscious knowledge" about internal states—homeostasis as far back as the cell itself where no brain resides! (p. 138)—and sees the evolution of the brain as permitting "the life urge to be regulated ever so effectively and, at some point in evolution, knowingly" (p. 139).

In the section under the heading "The Autobiographical Self and the Unconscious" (p. 226), Damasio recognizes the vital role of unconscious knowledge not only as splintered events—as the dissociative responses shown by face-agnosic patients who consciously are equally unable to cognitively recognize unknown and previously known faces while they show a distinct difference in skin conductance between the two sets of images[9]—but as the main system of brain dynamics eventuating also in conscious awareness. In

---

[7] The avoidance of any rapport between a dynamic unconscious and a dynamic core might rest on the uneasiness that Edelman and Tononi convey concerning the scientific validity of data collected through a different language from the one used by the objective observer. Or it might rest on some degree of unfamiliarity with the language of subjectivity.

[8] Biologically based epistemology considers consciousness to be a sine qua non of mental acts (Edelman & Tononi, 2000, p. 218).

[9] It appears that Edelman and Tononi (2000) were basically trying to explain dissociative phenomena when they advanced the proposal of splintered dynamic cores. Indeed, they appear

discussing the formation and the organization of memories that constitute the autobiographical self he points to the importance of the emotional valence and weight that is attached to these memories and how these attributes might lead the brain to process the mnestic structures differently. We are (usually) conscious of the contents of the experiences but not of the recording processes nor of their robustness and of the importance assigned to them. "Nor do we know how the contents become interrelated as memories and are classified and reorganized in the well of memory; how linkages among memories are established and maintained over time, in the dormant, implicit, dispositional mode in which knowledge exists within us" (Damasio, 1999, p. 226).

He distinguishes sets of memories that are easy to recall and routinely recalled in our daily trade with the experience of living (as our names and identity, orientation to time, space, persons, recent events, plans for the immediate future, and the like); and other sets that may remain unconscious for long periods, that may undergo a process of unconscious reorganization to a product that will differ from the original, or actually never emerge as conscious mental images.

> Instead, they may promote the retrieval of other memories which do become conscious in the form of other concrete facts or as concrete emotional states. In the extended consciousness of that moment, the facts ... may appear unmotivated, although a web of connections does indeed exist sub rosa, reflecting either the reality of some moment lived in the past or the remodeling of such a moment ... (p. 227)

Damasio's encompassing proposal of the unconscious is captured in his list of what it includes:

  I. all the fully formed images to which we do not attend;
  II. all the neural patterns that never become images;
  III. all the dispositions that were acquired through experience, lie dormant, and may never become an explicit neural pattern;
  IV. all the quiet remodeling of such dispositions and all their quiet renetworking—that may never become explicitly known; and
  V. all the hidden wisdom and know-how that nature embodied in innate, homeostatic dispositions.
  Amazing, indeed, how little we ever know. (p. 228)

To recapitulate the information on the unconscious expressed in the objective language of neuroscience, Edelman and Tononi offer a significant insight into the neurophysiology of large sets of unconscious data, as automatic behaviors, for which they propose in masterly detail neuroanatomical systems,

---

to classify all these phenomena as due to some "maladaptation." The trend is implicit even in their suggestion of a mechanism of repression causing such splinter systems to coexist in the unconscious (p. 190).

and to which the guiding rules of nonlinear science seem overall to apply as well. They appear less at ease with the interphase between the phenomenon of consciousness, as they envision it, and unconscious dynamics, and they tend to consider (all) manifestations of such interactions as deviant (splintered). Although their dynamic core appears to be a fitting neurobiological metaphor for the phase space, what I perceive as missing is the appreciation of emergence and of the ongoing interaction among the dynamics at different levels of description.

Damasio's model instead recognizes very clearly the immensity of the phase space out of which consciousness—and mind?—emerge; and recognizes the presence in such space not only of neural patterns but of mental patterns as well, in actual or in dispositional states: images that have been formed and images that have not yet been formed, but may be formed at any moment—a condition that reflects the hyperimmense dimension of creativity described in Chapter 2 (p. 24).[10] When superimposed upon each other, these two models offer a very valuable and comprehensive neurobiological perspective of the unconscious dimension of mind.

What can the language of the subjective experience, the first-person language, contribute to the discussion about unconscious structures of mind? The psychological sciences offer an abundance of theories, or metaphors, on these phenomena and their review is beyond the scope of this chapter. The myth of Psyche is very effective in illustrating the relationship between ego consciousness and unconscious operations of a routine type (a la Edelman) as well as of a more generalized and decisional type. Apuleius describes "voices" emerging from an unknown, invisible dimension, that not only address routine cyclic needs such as nourishment and sleep, but also inform the ego about the structure of the self and question her value systems and her limited knowledge. Furthermore, the entire dimension of Eros remains clouded in obscurity and wonderment, without precise definition, although Psyche can experience it deeply and be enriched by its input.

The subjective description by Apuleius reproduces, to be sure, his own particular version of the collective mythical understanding of the organization of mind and of the interaction between self and ego. I will now present a modern reenactment of the myth and by this means I will focus on indirect proofs of the unconscious participation in mental functioning—and of the content of ego consciousness; and I will concentrate not so much on routines

---

[10] I suspect that one reason for the difference between how these three scientists envision the unconscious rests on the fact that Edelman and Tononi may not conceive that mental patterns could exist outside of the state of consciousness, so that for them all that precedes such a functional state is exclusively a neural pattern without any intrinsic decisional capability. On the contrary, Damasio accepts the existence of unconscious mental images.

and subroutines as on decisional, meaningful processes that bring about the emergence of new insights.[11]

Let us consider the case of a hypothetical woman subject[12] who presented as a standing problem (and as the overt or covert cause for seeking psychotherapy) significant difficulties in her relationship to her partner (s): another Psyche disconnected from Eros. The way she may initially describe the difficulty—to herself and to the therapist—can be summarized as: .

> I need to stay away from him, he is bad for me.

If explored a little further, this initial presentation will evolve into (again summarized):

> look how many attributes he has that endanger my security and satisfaction.[13] I have to make him change and understand why he is bad for me and what makes him so.

As therapy probes at hidden themes, memories, and configurations of value systems, a progressive shift emerges in the conscious organization of mind that can be, for this particular subject, summarized as follows:

> I have to stay away from him because I feel bad about being close. Look how many attributes I projected on (attributed to) him that endanger my security and satisfaction. I have to change and understand what is going on inside of me that makes me feel this way about closeness.

The processes that had loaded the area of relatedness to the male with dysfunctionality, and the processes involved in the gradual change of that dysfunction were and are largely in the unconscious realm. The behavioral difficulties at this phase of therapy persist: she still perceives a freezing response, or anxiety, when attempting intimacy or trust. What has changed is the mental experience of the difficulty: he has become, somehow (!) "safe" and "desired" but internal factors continue to feed and oblige a dysfunctional response, although, apparently, with diminishing impact; "something," inside, is changing. Unknown factors related to retrievable or irretrievable experiences (fitting quite well Damasio's comments reported above) created in the past a

---

[11] I will return to the phenomenon of insight in Chapter 9, but I need to anticipate here that there is a substantial difference between a routine, or automatic behavior (old knowledge used to repeat the same task), and insight or intuition (old knowledge used to seek a new task and a new outcome).

[12] All the cases that I will discuss in this book represent clinical material that was exposed to intersubjective assessment (by the therapist), as was the case for all the clinical vignettes presented elsewhere (Sanguineti, 1999).

[13] I will discuss these terms in greater detail in Chapter 8. Basically, they reflect all that contributes to, or threatens, inner and outer harmony (or homeostasis).

distancing reflex that was in its own way adaptive in that it protected from traumatic memories, from pain, from unexplainable panic or fear.

However, as the hidden coping mechanism continued to direct overt behavior and to dictate the predominant, negative emotional valence attributed to relating to others, the absence and fear of relatedness and intimacy came to clash with the opposite, natural, evolutionary need to exist in a connected state (this natural developmental need for connectedness, expounded by Jessica Benjamin among others, will be revisited in Chapter 12).

The inner tension surfaced as generalized feelings of unhappiness and unfulfillment; these feelings were misattributed to other causes, such as jobs and partners' characteristics.[14] Eventually the inner strain became overtly symptomatic, with chronic irritability and self-doubts, and the emergence of somatic involvement as headaches, "heart palpitations" and episodic tachycardia, and a "nervous stomach." This scenario—the actual values and decisional choices underlying the vague affective and behavioral outcomes—operated in the self system, where the early experiences were still active and running; one could depict them as vast metastable neuronal assemblies, or as the attractor illustrated in Figure 2-3, that had become reinforced and prioritized because they carried an apparent survival value. The ego perceived the outcomes while developing a certain awareness of increasing discomfort, of the ineffectiveness of conscious attempted solutions, and of the absence from her life of the relatedness than she consciously wished she had.[15]

Security and satisfaction were no longer effectively protected and the need for a more radical "cure" became apparent. Incidentally, she described her resistance "to seek help"; a resistance that was very consistent with the scenario: the idea of therapy implied requirements for trust and intimacy with the stranger/therapist and therefore reverberated in a negative way at the center of the very problem it was supposed to address.

The process of change was explored and conducted through the ego. This process fed the self with new or revised information; mental images and neural patterns in the systems of assemblies carrying specific values and self-concepts underwent a gradual change as new meanings were attached to old *experiences*. The ego was still largely unaware of the process, although occasionally "informed" through dreams and intuitions,[16] but she "sensed" that "something" was going on inside of her.

---

[14] At this stage, this particular Psyche does not as yet feel forlorn and responsible for the "neglect"; she still feels that no partner is good enough or that the "right" partner has still to show up.

[15] Now she bears a close resemblance to the Psyche of old: she feels unwanted, undesirable, not fitting the "family" expectations; she becomes unhappy, depressed, and her life loses meaning.

[16] A similar process underlies the organization of a physiological intuition or "new idea" that sprouts out into consciousness. The phenomenon will be revisited in Chapter 9.

Indeed, the attributes of unconsciousness and invisibility with which the unconscious dynamics are traditionally characterized are not as rigid and complete as they have been depicted, particularly by the modern rational mind. "Something" transpires. What the conscious ego may perceive, if it gives sufficient attention, is the weight of the unconscious upon the overt organization of thought: local gravitational fields (Figure 2-3) become experienced, even if not yet "seen" as such, or very fleetingly at best. A subject who had misread (in a way consistent with a highly negative father transference) the affective content of a very marginal statement by the therapist (in a context that in a normal interaction would have been completely dismissed, as the subject easily recognized) left with some vague irritation, "not worth mentioning." As he was driving away the irritation grew; he then had "a flashing image, that came up from my unconscious, too fast to be fully retrieved, of a cowering child on the ground (and he reenacted the image by leaning backward and protecting his face with his arms) and a bellowing adult standing over him. It was so fast and it was gone; as those subliminal ads that they talk about." One is reminded of the comments advanced by Hebb (1949) on subliminal perception (previously reported, p. 59, *n.* 1).

One is also reminded of a similar state of affairs that characterized the field of astronomy. Of the entire mass of the universe, 80 percent is present as invisible matter. If the astronomers had relied solely on what they saw they would have built a model of a universe that would be much smaller than the actual one. However, they gradually became aware that certain phenomena, such as the orbits of the celestial bodies, did not perform in ways consistent with the Newtonian system of physical laws; they appeared to be affected by "something" that caused irregularities in their celestial behavior. Rather than dismissing these irregularities as odd events in an otherwise well-understood state of affairs, they were explored and it became clear that the major part of the universe is made up by dark matter, which is responsible for vast gravitational fields. The realization stimulated an entirely new area of research that eventually began to define not only the role but also the hypothetical composition of this dark matter.

Similarly, the language of the first-person experience is able to capture to some extent the weight effect of the dynamic unconscious upon the visible structure of mind and to suggest that such weight is considerable, therefore implying that these dynamics are (as Damasio insinuates) quite considerable as well.

If mental science continues, however, either to marginalize the role of unconscious dynamics upon the formation of ego consciousness, or to discard the data presented in the psychological language because they are considered "nonscientific," the science will inevitably end up with a very impoverished model of the mental universe.

To conclude, the three languages support each other in conveying specific information about the unconscious: the interactive and recursive dynamics through the levels of the cognitive hierarchy find correspondence in the reentrant mechanism and the dynamic core of Edelman (with the caveats noted earlier on); in the autobiographical self and the list of unconscious activities of Damasio; in the dynamic unconscious of modern psychology; in the "invisible servants"; and in Eros' presence that Apuleius describes as giving expression and meaning to the riches of Psyche's castle.

Chapter 7

THE DATABASE

What do the riches consist of? We have considered in the past two chapters how the brain organizes and stores information.[1] Are we in a condition to trace the categories of information that participate to the "libraries of knowledge" (Sanguineti, 1999, pp. xiv–xv) upon which our brain counts in the process of negotiating life? You will notice that the three languages address this issue from different perspectives; they should best be used to complement each other, rather than to enhance and confirm each other, as has been the case until now. Nonlinear science formulates the phase-space representing mind as holding a hyperimmense amount of data. These data are not specified by content but, as they pertain to all levels of the biological and cognitive hierarchies, they include categories that span from genetics to internal environment, to the personal psychophysical development, to the fields of society and culture.

Actually, nonlinear science is not so much concerned with which type of data is transmitted and stored in the human brain as it is with the self-sustaining relationships of causality that are active in the biological world at all levels of description. Consciousness and the human mind are just some of the myriad of systems observable in the biological world that are guided by the rules of nonlinear science; each one of these systems carries its own set of specific operative dynamics.[2] If the language of physical science makes a statement

---

[1] A review of the process of memory itself is beyond the scope of this book. Here we take memory as a given, one of the fundamental functions of brain and body: consider the memory of the immune system. Edelman discusses non-representational memory (Edelman & Tononi, 2000, p. 93) and Damasio describes autobiographical memory as a formative component of the autobiographical self (1999, pp. 17, 199).

[2] Interactions among systems complicate things further. Just consider the effect of climate on the psychological state (seasonal affective disorder representing a major example) as well as on physical aspects of the subject (aches and pains aggravated by cold damp weather being a common affliction); and the effect of culture and social forces on weather patterns (global warming and polar cap changes being extreme examples).

concerning the categories of data, it is that they probably comprise innumerable subsets in order to cover all possible combinations: a hyperimmense number of data organized in an innumerable number of subsets or categories.

The neurosciences offer, as we have seen, a description of how the data are organized and how they are operative, with structurally or functionally selected neural systems providing local processing, and generalized connective systems providing joint participation from the diverse zones of localized activity; the phenomena of reentry and the related processes of categorization and recategorization illustrate these neural mechanisms in depth.

The neurosciences, however, have less to say about the actual content of the data; they may differentiate the different sensory modalities because of the differences in the supporting neuroanatomy, and they emphasize the role of values (Edelman) and feelings (Damasio) in driving mental activity; however, the interest of these neuroscientific models rests primarily on how the brain operates the information it contains; naturally, the type of information processed will differentially affect neural interactions and outcome, but the modus operandi of the brain is not affected, per se.[3] The statement conveyed by the language of the objective observer is a statement about neurophysiological mechanisms that elucidate how the system is indeed capable of processing all these data in coherent and meaningful ways, and how this processing is actually carried out.

What can the first-person language offer concerning the content of the database? The language has actually dealt consistently and primarily with content: from the Egyptian metaphors onward the human subject has struggled with the overt and covert themes of mind, and this focused interest has colored most, if not all, psychological research, even at the cost of giving little or no attention to the actual functioning of the biological structure and inviting a separation between the realm of the neural and that of the mental. Nevertheless, the richness of information that emerged out of the inter-subjective work of therapy and from the theoretical analysis of the information (combined with the more limited speculations of philosophy) is quite substantial and it offers significant material, sufficient to propose a diagrammatic organization of some of the data into major subsets or categories that seem to reoccur with consistent regularity.

The data available through the first-person language are evidently formed only by mental images, bound into a representational memory. This set of data is retrievable exclusively through the language of the subjective experience, while the neural patterns that characterize nonrepresentational memory are

---

[3] To illustrate this point, consider how Edelman addresses the unconscious routines and subroutines. He hints to specific systems for each one of them but the modus operandi is similar, through parallel chains connecting the thalamo-cortical system to the cortical appendages.

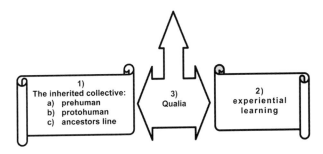

Figure 7-1: The three main libraries of knowledge.

accessible—*in their form, not in their meaning*—only through the language of objective neuroscience. Therefore all content that remains bound to neural patterns of processing—including the majority of the data dealing with internal homeostasis—will not be included in Figure 7-1. Apuleius describes how in the castle of Psyche an endless series of staterooms ("Fabrica perfecta," perfect structures) contain "all that was and is," a treasure that appears to be limited only by the future dimension of time. I have resorted to this metaphor used by Apuleius in order to address specifically the *content* of the psychological structure; I have renamed the staterooms and called them *libraries* and the treasure has become *knowledge*. The investigation of these libraries has been a major interest of mine, during the years that I have spent observing human minds gradually unfold their content within the psychotherapeutic scenario. This extended observation has provided significant information on the topic, which corroborated the abundant material collected and described by so many other intersubjective observers.

I have presented a detailed description of some orders of data in my work *Landscapes in My Mind* (1999), in which I correlated examples from personal experience with material derived from therapy. Therefore much of the information that follows will retrace the format followed in that book.

As illustrated schematically in Figure 7-1, we can observe three major categories of data:

1. The first library consists of inherited collective material, which has been a topic of great interest for evolutionary psychologists. Evolutionary psychology operates on the recognition that the human brain is adapted with a large collection of functionally specialized programs that evolved to solve the adaptive problems regularly encountered by our first ancestors.

The programs reflect adaptational coping attitudes with origins that date to long before the emergence of our ancestors, and which therefore are present also in other species. Because humans share a universal architecture, all ordinary individuals are endowed with the early evolutionary programs as well as the species-specific and culture-specific sets of preferences, motives, shared conceptual frameworks, emotion programs, and the like, that operate beneath the surface of expressed individual variability. Naturally, this view of human development requires that the evolutionary foundation be a solid reality (the same requirement applies to nonlinear science and it was addressed in Chapter 2). If one rejects the evolutionary theory or the set of physics guiding biological phenomena, then the entire interpretation crumbles. Personally, I have been utterly unable, despite strong efforts, to conceptualize life in a nonevolutionary way, even if my personal definition of evolution is rather unrestricted; it can even include variants like the "intelligent design" concept, because in my opinion these variants simply differ on the ultimate cause of it all (the Aristotelian final cause). It is difficult, without resorting to evolution, to explain impressive instances of shared characteristics such as the origin–recognition–complex (ORC) proteins that monitor or carry instructions for crucial episodes of cell mitosis and that are shared with yeasts and fruit. Origin–recognition–complex proteins are specific proteins that bind to sequences of the genome, and by stimulating the unwinding of the double helix, expose the DNA to the enzymes that copy it. In this way they induct the process of DNA replication. During the past decade, researchers identified well-defined origin sequences in yeast, and described several proteins that bind to these sequences (ORC). The genetic code for the complex was then tracked down and cloned, and this achievement allowed for a more precise exploration of its functions. Recent studies based on the use of cloned genetic material indicate that such codes have been maintained through evolution, so that they can be found in the yeast as well as in the fruit fly Drosophila and in humans. Furthermore, some of these studies also reported that the ORC gene of the fruit fly can replace certain functions of the same gene complex in the yeast, when inserted in a mutant form of the plant that has been made gene defective. The first forms of land plants are dated to the Silurian period, over 400 million years ago. The first organized, multicellular sea life can be traced back to over 500 million years ago. This may be how long these genetic instructions have been shared by the various species since they came into being. Other instructions may be very much older than these, as they may have been used and transmitted down the evolutionary path since the origin of life on Earth approximately 4 billion years ago.

We are reminded that so far as human beings are concerned, we are actually dealing with "an intellect a billion years old, in a body which is an ape on the back of a rat that grew out of a lizard. Can you imagine what comes out of the dark places, (when) uncontrolled?" (Pratchett, 2001, p. 336). The "evolutionary" library therefore contains three sets of interrelated "collections," a sort of historical record of life's walk through time.

- The prehuman collection includes information about evolutionary adaptation that preceded the differentiation of our genus Homo from its predecessors.

We share these data—mentalistic as well as physical—with other species. I have commented on the sexual phenotype earlier on, as an example of a continuous template that evolved out of prehuman sex-linked characteristics that differentiated the gender roles: it prized hormonally based male aggressivity and strength-based dominance to counterpoint an equally hormonally based female connectedness[4] and receptivity. The phenotype laid the foundation for the patriarchal template that provides the knowledge on which the brain acts. The experience of territoriality and the related adaptive signals that modulate competitiveness represent another instance of this type of data and are illustrated in Figure 7-2. Their emergence in different species is a strong indicator that they belonged to a common evolutionary pathway and were incorporated into various "branches" of the tree as these diverse species began to take form. The figure should help to dispel doubts about our prehuman core and its dynamic persistence in today's organization of mind. A strict behaviorist would be forced to conclude that the sets of minds represented in the figure are very closely related, if not practically identical, because of the strikingly close similarity in the behaviors. Indeed, the inheritance of ancient mentalistic programs makes as much sense as the inheritance of programs that direct the development of the physical self.[5] Just as we do not reinvent with each birth the programs for the formation of our limbs, so we do not reinvent the territorial response. We simply keep readapting an inherited template to our subjective experiences.

- A second collection of inherited knowledge contains data about the very early roots of the human mind: primal human evolution and the emergence of specific values and needs (Sanguineti, 1999, pp. 87–102).
- A third collection of genetic knowledge contains information about a narrower evolutionary sequence, which I have labeled the "ancestors' line." This line represents inherited favorite templates and data about a specific cultural niche and social structure, and related specific elaborations of primitive values and needs (Sanguineti, 1999, pp. 103–116).

In the example of the evolution of territoriality and dominance illustrated in Figure 7-2, the prehuman programs that had been used to convey the territorial message—and that had been transmitted from earlier forms of life, always under the rigid control of the genetic imperative—still persist in the depth of our brains, but have also developed into initially protohuman and then

---

[4] This speculative diversity in the neurohormonal and psychological development between genders will be revisited when discussing intersubjectivity and the position of Jessica Benjamin (1998).

[5] Other themes of emotional "recognition," of exploratory curiosity, of empathy for psychophysical distress that appear to cross the divide between species have been described elsewhere (Sanguineti, 1999, pp. 69–86).

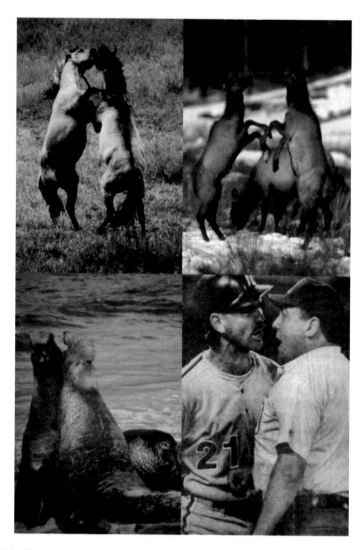

Figure 7-2: Territorial programs (counterclockwise from top right). A. Two Wapiti elk cows display for dominance, B. Two male Tarpan horses duel for control of a harem of mares. C. Dominance behavior among male elephant seals for the control of choice beaches. D. Dominance behavior in humans for control of the "sport hierarchy." Considering the vast differences among species, the behavior is strikingly similar, and it may indicate that the common path followed by the territorial programs was quite narrow. (Figure 7-2A: photography by D. J. Cox. Figure 7-2B: photograph by Tony Bomford. Both reproduced with permission by Oxford Scientific Films. Figure 7-2C; photograph by Frans Lanting; reproduced with permission by Minden Pictures. Figure 7-2D photo and photomontage by author.)

truly human and cultural internalizations of the concept of *territory* and of *dominance*. The first symbol came to include not only a strictly geographical message but also and predominantly a conceptual significance (consider the political, academic, financial territories, among the endless available list), while for the other symbol there was a gradual shift from dominance based primarily on physical strength and fighting experience, as in the case of the dominant buck, to dominance in task mastery and task hierarchy.

Echoing Mansfield (2000, p. 67) a contemporary summary of the territorial (and sexual) imperatives sees male heroism as expressed when the territory is safely sealed and its ownership assured, the enemies slain, the motives and values of the hero known and accepted, and the world finally reordered along the lines of the hero's vision (though not the Greek hero, however). Today's world offers very powerful examples of the reactivation of this dark hero figure.

2. The second library that contributes to our global knowledge comprises our experiential learning; this library contains all that we experience during an individual lifetime. These data are processed through the data from the first library, and the two sets constantly reclassify and reorganize each other. This interactive process is responsible for the exquisitely subjective and ever-changing characteristics of our minds.

3. The third major library contains affective information (I dedicate the next chapter to affectivity and its role). The common theme is that a shared attribute of the myriad of data outlined above is their being weighted with affective elements or *qualia*.[6] *Affectivity* is used in this context as a technical term that defines a family of states and events for which a "feeling" characteristic represents a primary attribute of each state. Affectivity and affective resonance constitute a communal pathway to the workings of the mind.

Perhaps at this time we need to redefine the term freedom as we redefined the term *consciousness*. I have a strong suspicion that Rousseau's position was very brave, but that his truly "free" individual, an intrinsic individuality of the self, is a dubious concept at best. "Fixed and universal values ignore the complexity, plurality, inconsistency and ambiguity of subjectivity, imprisoning us in the apparent duty of being a stable, fixed and authentic self" (Mansfield, 2000, p. 95). We ultimately cannot be free of the ecological niche because we are in symbiosis with the world and intrinsically intertwined in it, despite all our protestations to the contrary. This symbiosis applies not only to the biological hierarchy but also to the cognitive domain of culture, language, and the like. Even at the highest levels of the cognitive hierarchy we can move from culture to culture but we cannot move out of culture in any intrinsic way.

---

[6] The specific meaning that I attach to this term—and that differs from the common usage—will be clarified in the next chapter as well.

To conclude: the language of nonlinear dynamics supports and suggests that the information present within a mind, and participating to the process of thought production, is hyperimmense and dynamically connected. The third-person language of the objective observer identifies a neural system of sufficient structural and functional complexity to support the vast matrix of interactive data postulated by this system of physics. The language of the first-person experience describes the content and principal types of data in a very rich, highly documented, and consistent way, from the ancient mythical dimension to the modern array of psychological research. In the presentation of the findings from my research I have purposefully refrained from pointing to the similarities between these findings and those of many different schools of psychology. The similarities are nevertheless very visible; this is quite reassuring and offers a confirmation that this language, too, can offer a robust replicability within the variability imbued in the heterogeneous nature of all the samples that become the subject of investigation.

Chapter 8

AFFECTIVITY

The emotional dimension[1] has long been recognized as a cardinal aspect of mind and it has carried profound meaning through all the different metaphors that have been used to illustrate it. Damasio (1999) ultimately refers to it as the feeling of what happens, while Gelernter (1994) calls it the muse in the machine, and Apuleius (170 CE), reflecting the Greek mythical version, represents it as Eros.

I have indicated in the preceding chapter that nonlinear science is not so much concerned with the specifics of biological phenomena as it is with the self-sustaining relationships of causality that are active in the biological world. Its function is to provide parameters on which to assess the feasibility of the particular biological phenomenon that is under investigation. The parameters facilitate, however, a new conceptualization of affectivity, although they are not set out by the science expressly to illustrate it. Along these lines, I refer you to Figure 2-3 to exemplify how value systems and other stable emotional structures might act as local attractors and exercise constraints upon the modulation of neuronal assemblies and the direction of specific trains of thought.

Edelman has a limited input in the areas of affectivity, aside from the crucial role that he invests in the value systems. He assumes that "phenomenal states or qualia (sensations, raw feels, and the like, constituting collectively 'what it feels like to be an X') all exist in conscious humans" (1989, p. 24) and that these events are describable in third-person terms. He labels this position "the qualia assumption." In a brief review on affective disorders he comments on Carroll's (1993, pp. 163–186) theoretical suggestion that affective disorders (depression

---

[1] As mentioned earlier on, I use the term *affectivity* in a technical sense to define a family of psychic states and events for which a "feeling" characteristic represents a primary attribute of each state. It accommodates emotional constructs, affects, instincts, values, meanings, intentional states, and qualia.

and mania) may be due to dysfunctions in central systems governing pleasure-reward, pain regulation, and psychomotor facilitation. He comments that consciousness per se is not modified, but that disturbances in the "hedonic drive" may affect "the patient's conscious evaluative capacities" (Edelman, 1989, pp. 228–331).

In a more recent writing (1992), Edelman mentions components of the affectivity family:

> Feelings are a part of the conscious state and are the processes that we associate with the notion of qualia as they relate to the self: They are not emotions, however, for emotions have strong cognitive components that mix feelings with willing and with judgment in an extraordinarily complicated way. Emotions may be considered the most complex of mental states or processes insofar as they mix with all other processes. (Edelman, 1992, p. 176)

The qualia assumption achieves even greater depth and complexity in the more recent book by Edelman and Tononi (2000). They note:

> The qualia assumption states that the subjective, qualitative aspects of consciousness, being private, cannot be communicated directly through a scientific theory that, by its nature, is public and intersubjective... qualia can be considered forms of multidimensional discrimination that are carried out by a complex brain. No description can take the place of the individual subjective experience of conscious qualia. (Edelman & Tononi, 2000, p. 15)

Feelings per se are not mentioned, but, as we have seen, the value systems grow to assume a primary role. "Value systems and emotions are essential to the selectional workings of the brain that underlie consciousness" (p. 218).[2] One needs to keep in mind that these authors, as we discussed in Chapter 5, operate along a model that has consciousness as its sole objective, and HOC (conscious of being conscious) as the frontrunner.

Edelman's constraint when dealing with feelings finds its countermeasure in Damasio's primary concern with the affective dimension; the title, *The Feeling of What Happens* (1999), is by itself very descriptive of this neuroscientist's position. Affectivity permeates the search for consciousness and represents a primary force in the unconscious domain of neurodynamics as well.

Damasio considers all emotions as depending on innate brain devises laid down by a long evolutionary history, which are then fine-tuned by culture and by learning. All emotions share a common biological core characterized by: (1) a collection of specific chemical and neural responses; (2) the presence of a regulatory role seeking favorable life conditions; (3) biologically determined processes; (4) a restricted range of subcortical regions; (5) the capacity to be

---

[2] This is the only place where the term *emotion* appears. They are considered "fundamental both to the origins of and the appetite for conscious thought."

engaged automatically without conscious effort; (6) the use of the body as their theater while also intricately affecting brain operations involved in the organization of neural patterns as well as mental images. Overall, Damasio strongly promotes the concept that the affective domain assists the organism in *maintaining life*.

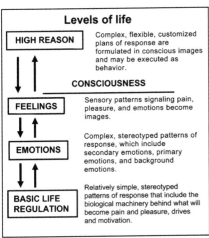

Figure 8-1: An affective hierarchy (modified from Antonio Damasio with permission by the Author. From *The Feeling of What Happens: Body and Emotion in the Making of Consciousness*, Harcourt Trade Publishers, 1999, p. 55).

Figure 8-1 illustrates the hierarchical order of affective states promulgated by Damasio; here he positions emotions and at least some "feelings"[3] below the separator of consciousness: an interesting view, that suggests how a significant part of the organization and role of affectivity happens in the unconscious.

I have already presented this author's articulation of mind and consciousness (self-consciousness as well as ego consciousness) as percolating upward through a sea of feelings. I will close this review of the information about affectivity that has emerged from the field of neuroscience by briefly mentioning some specific experimental research on affectivity that deals with unconscious recognition of emotions and with their role, as alerting systems, in directing adaptive and maladaptive behavior.

Kaszniak researched in depth specific conscious and unconscious aspects of emotions (1999). He has explored how these concepts might illustrate the search for homeostasis that could represent the core function of affectivity. Research in his lab with human subjects suggested that the subjective experience of emotions is guided, among other factors, by a valence dimension and an arousal dimension.

The valence dimension indicates the pleasure-displeasure weight that the brain allocates to a specific stimulus; it is reliably linked to facial muscles

---

[3] If I understand Damasio correctly, feelings represent mental patterns; they are, in a way, the self *experiencing* the neural emotional patterns and giving them a label of sorts.

electromyography (EMG), heart rate, and startle eye blink, and it finds further support in electroencephalographic (EEG) studies that show differential hemispheric involvement in positive and negative emotions. The arousal dimension indicates the level of emotional content or experience that a stimulus has to generate in order to elicit a response as expressed through EEG or skin conductance changes. Further experimental research with unmasked and masked stimuli indicates that both arousal and valence can be subjectively experienced in the absence of conscious awareness of the stimulus.

To conclude, the neuroscientific models used in this book offer diversified views on affectivity: from the vast affective model of Damasio to the constrained input of Edelman, framed by his focus on consciousness and on the qualia assumption, all these views emphasize the centrality of this family of dynamics in the neural and mental organization of mind.

Perhaps this is the best moment to digress and discuss the issue of qualia and the traditional meaning given to this term as contrasted to my specific meaning. In its traditional philosophical usage the term *qualia* describes, or is used to try to describe, simple sensations, the classic mantra usually being "the redness of red or the blueness of blue": that special subjective feeling that makes "red" red and not blue. Actually, neuroscientists are rather broad based about the consistent usage of this term. Damasio does not say much about qualia. He defines them as "the simple sensory qualities to be found in the blueness of the sky or the tone of sound produced by a cello" (1999, p. 9) and considers them as fundamental components of the images in his movie-in-the-brain metaphor. They belong to all those structures that "operate within the nonverbal vocabulary of feelings" (p. 313).

Edelman and Tononi give much more attention to the matter. They too introduce qualia as the redness of red and the blueness of blue; however, they proceed to explore them at greater depth; they assert that no theory or description can substitute for the individual's experience of a quale, and they go on to say that "each differentiable conscious experience represents a different quale, whether it is primarily a sensation, an image, a thought, or even a mood and whether, in retrospect, it appears simple or composite"; "each quale corresponds to a different state of the dynamic core, which can be differentiated from billions of other states within a neural space comprising a large number of dimensions" (Edelman & Tononi, 2000, p. 157).

They seem to conclude that everything conscious is a quale when they describe how:

> Contrary to common usage ... *every different conscious state deserves to be called a quale,* from the state of perceiving pure red, pure darkness, or pure pain, to the state of perceiving a complicated visual scene, and to the state of "thinking of Vienna," ... In short, a "pure" sensation of red defines a point in (a) *N*-dimensional state space as much as the conscious perception of a busy street in NYC, full

of different objects, sounds, smells, associations, and reflections, defines another
point. In both cases, the meaning of the conscious perception is given by the
discrimination among billions of other possible states of the core, each of which
would lead to different consequences. (p. 168)

This statement makes it difficult for me to differentiate between a quale and
consciousness, or even between a quale and the entirety of mind. It offers a very
close reformulation in neural terms of the multidimensional mental phase space
that we encountered in Chapter 2, given that, at least as I understand it, these
complex qualia represent instances of dynamic core *activation*. However, the
majority of the causal loops eventuating in the busy street in New York City
are not conscious events, even while we consciously perceive the emergent
outcome of their ongoing dynamics. Actually, we do not *really* perceive the
entire composite quale that Edelman and Tononi describe. Much if not most of
it is "subliminal"; and yet, all these other events are qualia in Edelman's sense
of the word.[4]

Faced with such a latitude in the conceptualization of qualia—including
philosophers, and it is sufficient to compare Searle (1992) with Dennett (1991)
to prove this point—I will stick to my use of the term *qualia*, which I have
consistently considered as the quanta of the mental domain. After all, no one
has a monopoly on language and we are all entitled to assign specific meanings
to words we use, provided we do so in a consistent fashion.

In my framework, qualia represent units of feeling.[5] Their primary domain
is the unconscious; their composite elaborations belong to both domains.
Actually, the conscious-unconscious divide is really not an issue here, and
probably it is not an issue for mental images in general as well. Functionally,
qualia are the *emotional qualifiers* of the contribution to my security and
satisfaction intrinsic to a specific state of affairs.

I use these terms in the sense given to them by H. S. Sullivan (1953); by *security* he meant the state acquired through the prevention or protection from
tension associated with the personal environment; by *satisfaction* he meant the
state acquired through the prevention or relaxation of tension from specific
inner drives. I have always found them to be very well-chosen psychological
definitions of the drives that directed the entire process of evolution.

In the biological organism these two sets of functions may have evolved
initially into "memories" of physical sensory experiences and then into psychological constructs, and consequently the latitude of their meaning has

---

[4] It may also be that these neuroscientists are "naive" to the complexity of emotional states and
they deal with the issue primarily as objective observers and from a logical, rational viewpoint,
or within the constraints of a laboratory situation.

[5] Physicist Nick Herbert liked to consider my qualia as quanta of subjectivity.

mushroomed. The mind processes everything along survival themes and analyzes whether any specific state of affairs presents adaptive (favorable) or maladaptive (unfavorable) potential to the organism's security and satisfaction.

The composite outcome of the affective valences intrinsic in each quale correlates with the "emotional valence" concept described by Kaszniak and directs the choice for the type of planned response (either approach or withdrawal). The final "global" feeling experience then activates action execution whenever it reaches a critical threshold. This final experience correlates with the "arousal" concept of emotions. Instincts, meanings, needs, and values possibly stem from the search for a more versatile and differentiated expression of the original drives. The progressive expansion and fine-tuning of the "qualia mesh" allowed for life to move from the fixed and mindless genetic programs, with the development of an organ of choice and reelaboration of alternatives (the brain). This evolutionary progression may look somewhat like this: Instinct → Quale → Aggregate of qualia → State of emotion → State of feeling → State of feeling made conscious.

An unusual contribution to the dimension of feelings, discussed from the perspective of artificial intelligence, but written in the language of the first-person experience, is offered by computer scientist David Gelernter, and I present it here as a fitting introduction to the subjective view of affectivity. A leading figure in computer science, Dr. Gelernter is one of the seminal thinkers in the field of parallel computing and he proposes an interesting angle to the relationship between affect and cognition, with specific reference to the link between artificial intelligence and affectivity. In his 1994 book (which carries the subtitle *Computerizing the Poetry of Human Thought*) he discusses at great length the role of affect in generating thought and in determining the type of thought processes, and goes on to discuss the relationship between affect and creativity.

He proposes a broad and continuous spectrum of ways to think that depends on the level of mental focus active at that specific time. In his words, "mental focus might sound like another way of saying 'degree of alertness'; what's new is the way *cognition as a whole* changes in response to changing focus" (p. 4). These changes are related to differences in the affective participation in the train of thoughts. Gelernter proposes that unexpected associations and transitions, and leaps in the thinking process, are due to an affective correlation between the overtly disparate components. "*Affect linking*, I will claim, is responsible for bringing these leaps about" (p. 6).

Two broad categories of mental focus are proposed, which represent the poles of a continuum:

- The *high focus band* at the top of the spectrum is characterized by a mode of thinking that is the ground for rationality and for all analytical and penetrating, sustained thinking activities among which are science, mathematics, engineering; it is the type that is simulated on a computer; it provides a powerful tool for problem-solving and is certainly very adaptive; it is unfeeling, or emotionally monochromatic, and the unfeeling aspect excludes distractibility and interferences, but it excludes also intuition and creativity and spirituality. In summary, "high-focus thought centers on two related mental acts: *honing in* and *suppressing individual idiosyncrasies in favor of common features*" (p. 76). High focus will never allow us to see all the experiences that are stored in memory because in this state affect linking is kept to a minimum or utterly suppressed.

- In the *low band of focus* mental leaps between apparently unrelated thoughts begin to emerge; these unexpected transitions are based on affect linking and are the ground for metaphorical, analogic thinking and creativity (I will revisit Gelernter's lines of reasoning about creativity in Chapter 9). "Low-focus streams aren't random; they are thematic; but their themes are emotional themes" (p. 32). The drawing of analogies is not computable and this entire mode of thinking is not computable as well. How analogical thinking works is still unknown.[6] He suggests that subjects may be differentially gifted with a palette of emotional responses (alexythymia being an extreme of a totally blank palette), where a highly nuanced palette stands for emotional acuity, this state correlating with high scores on the existing tests of creativity (p. 191).

It is also interesting to hear what this computer scientist has to say about emotions and computers: "The first step in a computer model of mind ought to be a computer model of the cognitive spectrum. If we don't know how to build such a model, we have no idea how a truly convincing fake mind would actually work" (p. 45). And again: "Creativity can only emerge, I believe, as a byproduct of affect linking in low-focus thought, and no existing computer program has ever grappled with low-focus thought." He concludes, however, that in his opinion these thought models are testable, in some different sense from what we now mean; the "high-focus 'experience-based deduction'... can be formalized" (p. 191) and the low-focus thought streams could eventually be formalized as well. He even anticipates "a formal logistic system that captures the notion of 'intuitive leaps' "(p. 191).

What does the research in the first-person language say about affectivity? The richest information on affectivity as a mental experience is written in the first-person language, which at present appears to be the only language fit to

---

[6] Gelernter points to the difference between convergent (or problem-solving or logical) and divergent (or analogical) thinking; test results for the first type tally well with the results of intelligence tests while divergent thinking does not; and these results should make us careful about our understanding of intelligence tests in general.

grasp and describe these phenomena. The neuroscientists cited above convey this message very clearly; indeed, their proposals are full of introspective resonance: their language and the concepts they use are imbued with a "feeling of knowing"[7] that to me is in itself an illustration of how their research and writings reflect also their unique "movement of the heart."[8]

At the beginning of our path to discovery we find the story of Psyche and Eros. Its crucial theme is the polarity between the beautiful but sterile Psyche (logos) and the creativity-inducing but obscure domain of Eros, and the story captures in a very evocative way the same polarity between rationality and affectivity described by Gelernter. Although the metaphors have changed, the content has not, including the focal spectrum: the sleeping condition of the myth correlates quite precisely with the dimming of consciousness necessary to enter a low-focus condition.

The entire myth is centered on the interplay between these two aspects of mind. The first "act" is concerned with the functional limitations of a consciousness that, being disconnected from its affective side,[9] responds in a chameleonlike fashion to affective experiences. Psyche is confronted with a multiplicity of emotional states while being herself "empty" of affective resonance, so that she is unappealing despite the attractiveness of her "visible" attributes, and unequipped to deal with the dimension of feelings. The ensuing struggle that forms the context of the myth is carried on between an intricate web of conflicting emotions that all compete to dictate specific, affect-linked behaviors, and a state of consciousness, metaphorically split off from its inner "riches," whose reasoning power and perception of reality shifts along with the prevailing emotion of the moment. (In Chapter 13 I will explore how this individual condition is also replicated in the dimensions of society and culture.) When she feels unconnected to the world she reverberates with her

---

[7] Consider the qualia "street of New York" image that Edelman and Tononi use. It is redolent of personal experience, some of which we can perceive in ourselves as a feeling of familiarity and connectedness. Through and behind this first layer, though, I can also grasp a set of poorly formed affective speculations and images of mine, concerning the mind that created the picture, while it was experiencing what is described. Something indefinite percolates, possibly through the choice and sequence of images and words, favored upon others. Truly, images often seem to reflect, in some mysterious way, not only "what is known" but also the "self in the act of knowing," as the psychotherapeutic movement has come to appreciate.

[8] As an illustrative reinforcement of the influence of affectivity upon science I repeat the statement by Wallace mentioned earlier: "What we really believe to be true will invariably influence what we believe to be of value; conversely, all of us, including scientists, seek to understand those aspects of reality that we value. Thus, the scientific world-view has been generated by the kinds of values and ideals held by the scientists. The mutual interdependence of values and beliefs is inescapable" (Wallace, 2000, p. 7).

[9] A case of "inner alexythymia": the inability to consciously experience its own emotional states.

own devaluation as she experiences it in others; when her first experience of low-focus thinking (Zephyr's calming lift and subsequent sleep) creates an "unexpected connection" (Gelernter, 1994, p. 86) to the previously unknown richness within her (the dimension of the palace), she is surprised and cannot trust her own intuitive power.[10] When she is met by the full affective expression of Eros she responds with eroticism and budding creativity, only to shift to fear and aversion when the jealousy and envy of her sisters load her mental image of the unseen Eros with their negative qualia; and she still cannot accept the fact that the majority of the experience in encountering one's own affectivity operates "out of the light of day," in the invisible domain of the unconscious. The second act of the tale will see Psyche's journey to search for a personal resolution of her condition and to assert her right to a permanent relationship with her emotional domain experienced by the ego with greater easiness and clarity, and I will return to it in Chapter 12.

Moving forward along the path, the clinical psychotherapeutic domain is saturated with illustrations of the ongoing central role of complex affective constructs—conscious as well as unconscious—in directing thought processes and behaviors (for a comprehensive exploration of the "qualia web," see also Sanguineti, 1999, pp. 117–134). Indeed, the entire psychoanalytic literature, irrespective of school of thought, concurs on the premise that the uninterrupted role of affectivity in thought and behavior represents the fundamental tenet for psychic functioning.[11] Human activity—from major events carrying worldwide effects to slips of the tongue and daily rituals—is a compromise emerging from a multidimensional dynamic phase space of instinctual derivatives (the qualia web); or from an extremely intricate network of neural connectivity, modulated by and processing systems of values and inputs from specific emotional brain areas; or from the interplay between Eros (libido?) and Logos; or from the outcome of the interaction between the conscious subject and numinous manifestations spinning out of other realms of experience (religion and myth). Choose your preferred metaphor. A healthy evolution of mind postulates the gradual integration, and mastery, into ego consciousness of the products from the affective cauldron, with the understanding that its myriad of dimensions could never be fully contained and known within the domain of the ego.

This state of affairs finds regular confirmation from clinical material. Quite often the emotional pull—the weight factor mentioned in Chapter 6— is perceived distinctly at the conscious level, although the emotional content is

---

[10] Gelernter (1994, p. 100) makes an interesting comment when he reflects that "not every affect link reveals a fact of scientific value, or of any practical value, but every affect link reveals a truth" a personal truth concerning that specific mental universe and its own rules and systems of values directing its personal survival.

[11] Starting with Freud's brilliant insight that for memory traces to be stored they require affective loading.

hidden. For a particular patient, PD, the words *going South* (and *going North*) had come to assume a very intricate, multidimensional meaning by associating concrete "geographical" events with a specific behavioral pattern that would surface, under different disguises, in many aspects of his life. He was very aware that the "going south" became operative *under the pressure of a distinctly felt affective injunction*; however, he could not discriminate the content of the emotional package. He was only aware of the strong arousal dimension intrinsic in the emotional aggregate, when it became activated into ego consciousness.

Another subject, TP, described with significant pride a conscious structure that considered any emotional manifestation as "silly" and not worth the expenditure of psychic energy; poetry, romance, songs, and impressionistic art were a waste of time and shallow endeavors, compared with philosophy and logic, mathematics, symphonic music (and cerebral jazz), and architectural design. Unerringly in high focus, he presented a highly organized pattern of speech, and a powerful logical articulation of his train of thought that left him always firmly in control. The only problem consisted in recurring episodes of significant depression; but even at those times he maintained an outwardly unchanged affective facade. The "depression" was an unformed and indistinct mood state, highly unpleasant and paralyzing. Actually, there was no sense that this state was a "mood" or had any relationship with the type of filtered emotions that he had intermittently allowed himself to experience. Depression was simply a "profound heaviness," a "bad condition to be in."

The dismantling of the high-focus apparatus, required in order to facilitate channels of communication with the emotional domain, was a very hard project because anything experienced as a loss of control was quite unpalatable to the ego. When this was achieved and unexpected associations (and dreams!) began to float around, he found that his obsession with logic and control was partially an "inherited" (paternal) mode of being, but primarily its roots consisted of devastating exposures to emotional dyscontrol that he had experienced in his very early life. These experiences obligated the high-focus pattern of living as the only defensive operation that appeared sufficiently adaptive and that could counterbalance his abysmal sense of personal danger, failure, and loss of control. Exposed to wild and scary emotions during his early development, and obligated for his own survival to eliminate any retaliatory urge that he might have felt, he came to see emotions as dangerous and destructive psychological states that had to be avoided at all costs; the most effective defense was the complete elimination of his own affectivity. The defense required a full absorption into abstract thinking and hard science, and the avoidance of all those social interactions that might activate any feeling response which could then make him exposed and vulnerable.

In other scenarios, complex affective memories may remain linked in the unconscious with early kinesthetic experiences and eventuate in unexpected connections between the two realms, one component of the link emerging into consciousness as a somatic event (refer to the correlation between masked memories and somatic markers described by Kaszniak) while the mental affective images remain hidden.

Psychotherapy is rich in examples of these phenomena. Apart from classical clinical conditions as varied as asthma, type A personality, hypertension and cardiomyopathies, vaginismus, gastrointestinal syndromes, and teeth grinding or full temporomandibular joint syndrome (TMJ), transitory unexpected (and often eventually recognized as maladaptive) physical responses are common events: if an individual carries emotional, unconscious ("forgotten")[12] mental images and kinesthetic memories of inflicted pain, then the exposure of the body-self to the potentiality for a vulnerable state will not infrequently activate defensive body responses, *even if the current situation is considered "safe" and even desirable to the ego*: muscular tensing up, cutaneous zones of heightened sensitivity or actual hyperesthesia to touch, tachycardia, vertigo, nausea, urinary urgency, erectile failure, the list can be quite long.

Affectivity has been perceived since ancient times as the driving force behind human behavior, inclusive of inner thought processes as well as outwardly directed actions. This view finds confirmation and support in modern neuroscientific models: from the value systems of Edelman and Tononi to Damasio's feeling of what happens, and to the muse *not* in the machine of Gelernter. In the language of nonlinear physics the various manifestations of this family of neural and mental patterns may be conceptualized as rather stable attractors, as a myriad of points in the phase space of mind (or in the multidimensional space of the dynamic core, or in the dynamic unconscious) that put their ever-constant and ever-changing constraints upon the emergent trains of thought, through self-sustaining loops at multiple levels of the hierarchies.

---

[12] This state of affairs invites a discussion on the "false memories" syndrome, that actually belongs to this book only in a marginal way. I just want to point out that "memories" in a strict psychological sense are simply idiosyncratically stored personal experiences whose relationship to actual reality is approximate at best, in a way consistent with Edelman's message that we *categorize reality by value*. And we need to remind ourselves all the time how actually multidimensional "values" are, reflecting as they do their percolation through the entire sets of the libraries of knowledge. The more the subjective affective loading attached to an experience is, the more the "objective" external reality to which the experience relates may differ from our recollection of it. Still, psychologically speaking, those memories are true to the experience as it was lived through by the subject.

Chapter 9

THE NEURAL/MENTAL GAP: INTUITION, SELF AND EGO, A TRILINGUAL MAP

Aristotle defines imagination as the movement that results from an actual sensation. In other words, it is the process by which an impression of the senses is pictured and retained before the mind, and is accordingly the basis of memory. The representative pictures that it provides form the materials of reason. Illusions and dreams are both alike due to an excitement in the organ of sense similar to that which would be caused by the actual presence of the sensory phenomenon. Memory is defined as the permanent possession of the sensuous picture as a copy that represents the object of which it is a picture. Recollection, or the calling back to mind the residue of memory, depends on the laws that regulate the association of our ideas. We trace the associations by starting with the thought of the object present to us, then consider what is similar, contrary, or contiguous.

The creation of images out of the matter of neural cells has been and is an event that deeply captures human curiosity while continuing to elude it. I mentioned earlier how Voltaire, in more recent times, has described a thought as an image that paints itself upon the brain. Modern neuroscience and modern psychological science are still basically at this level of description when trying to explain how neuronal activity becomes a mental image. The information gathered by reading the tale in the three languages, however, allows us at least to safely propose that the painting is organized in the unconscious, possibly initially in neural patterns that could be theoretically recorded and analyzed from the third-person perspective, and then in mental patterns that may eventually be translated into consciousness as emergent outcomes; at this point the painting can be consciously grasped, but exclusively from the first-person perspective. We are still stuck with the fact that the "brain-mind complex"[1] appears to operate in two domains: the biological and the cognitive.

---

[1] The term in my opinion is overall an ugly and somewhat hypocritical image, that expresses the confusion and discomfort about siding with one way or the other. It is the product of the lack

Figure 9-1 represents in diagrammatic form a schema for the creation of the painting. This figure builds on Figure 7-1, which illustrates the database participating in the formation of the brain's global knowledge. The libraries of global knowledge, which represent vast multidimensional, nonlinear dynamic configurations, are activated and tapped into by the requirements arising from our interaction with classical reality—high-focus, rational, problem-oriented, scientific thinking, with its own requirements, is included in this reality. The requested material becomes organized into a representational construct that could be recognized by us and by others, and could be applied to the state of affairs it pertains to. These representational configurations are what HOC is made of and represent the language and content of the ego. Elsewhere (Sanguineti, 1999, pp. 33–34) I labeled these two configurations as very rapid thinking (or VRT) and relational thinking (RT).

The labels are admittedly rather plain and terribly unscientific, but they try to convey the point that both are a type of "thinking", not only electrochemical neural noises. I have repeatedly hinted at my notion that we are the inevitable products of our interactive history. The development of the brain found its causality (all of it, from material to final) in the enhancement of the channels for information exchange and in the elaboration of choices fundamental to such interactive processes throughout the evolutionary dynamics that guided the emergence of mankind. Furthermore, humanity is a classical reality object: while at some arcane level we might share with the basic elemental structures of the universe in exotic ways and energy fields, the entire selectional process that

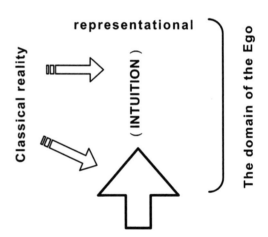

Global knowledge, non representational, in neural and mental patterns, under ongoing nonlinear revision...

Figure 9-1: The emergence of images in ego consciousness.

---

of fit between brain science and mind science, of the attempts to give both metaphors an equal share of attention, and to avoid the risk of being labeled "mental" or "biological." I personally would prefer to use the term brain with the proviso that concerning mental phenomena I am a property dualist of sort, possibly due to ignorance.

supported the emergence of the species and our own *meaningful* existence has been acted out in the macro-field of classical reality. More precisely, the entire selectional process has been acted out *in the interaction*[2] between us as subjects and classical reality.[3] Along with Kristeva (1982) we may come to agree that the boundary around subjectivity is never finished; the object and the subject are never absolutely distinct, and therefore subjectivity never quite stabilizes but is an ongoing system, evocative of the recategorization process described by Edelman and of the positive feedback systems of nonlinear science.

Differences in the intensity of attention focused upon the "classical reality" task regulate differences in the type of emergent products (for an exhaustive discussion on the topic see Sanguineti, 1999, pp. 53–68). When the focus is high and the train of thought is narrowed to the task and "converges" in a problem-solving mode, unexpected associations are filtered out and the "task-into-ego-consciousness" sequence becomes a prevailing attractor operating in that specific phase space. Logical linearity assumes a definite directing quality; rules are substituted by laws, and singularity by stochastic ensembles. The phenomenon of emergence is not perceived because it is implicitly anticipated and taken for granted; there are neither distracting nor surprising responses surfacing from the deep.

The risk from traveling such a narrow path resides in the very numbness of the process. If the machinery gets stuck it will keep grinding its wheels upon the same tracks, and eventually sputter and stall. This is such a well-known and well-described phenomenon that it does not require further examples.

The answer to the question as to what guides the translation of the selected constructs that emerge into conscious awareness, points to that process variously called analogic thinking, insight, intuition (Apuleius describes the phenomenon as "voices without a body, invisible servants").

Intuition consists in the use of old knowledge, located out of conscious awareness, to seek a new task and a new outcome, without any apparent participation from the ego. With the dimming of focus the "intuitive" mechanism assumes a sharper configuration than in high focus, and it is easily perceived as such. In the case of a task for which a solution is not forthcoming, "intuition" appears as the sudden emergence of such a solution—or of a new path toward it—without any conscious awareness of the processes involved. In other instances (such as therapy) the intuitive process is characterized by the

---

[2] The importance of realizing that the subject is essentially an interactive structure cannot be overemphasized and will become even clearer when I discuss the transference—countertransference themes.

[3] This can consist in the flight of a bird, the unfolding of a synaptic vesicle, the neuromodulation of a value, a busy street in New York City, a thought process, the feeling of a happening, a touch, a mathematical formula, Guernica, hunger.

unexpected shift in the associational chain. The bridge is an affective link, to use Gelernter's perceptive insight (!). At low focus—the lowest being states like sleep—the brain works on whole memories rather than fine details, where *"the character of the memory as a whole* is subtly captured by the feeling it evokes, by its *emotional content"* (p. 78). This way of thinking fosters creativity, from the normal, garden variety to the type expressed by a chess master or by the unpredictable "jumps" of a genius, or of a psychotic state. Silvano Arieti, once called the father of schizophrenia because of his profound analysis of the syndrome, pointed to a certain similarity between the thought processes of a schizophrenic and that of a genius, in that both minds are not rigidly anchored to logical reality but can "follow" unexpected connections among realms apparently unrelated to each other. He proposed that when human responses are mediated by cognitive processes "they generally follow the mechanisms that in Freudian theory are ascribed to the *secondary process* [and that] correspond to ordinary logical thinking" (Arieti, 1967, p. 328). Creativity allows for a degree of freedom from the ordinary secondary process mode. The *process* of creativity (not the *product*) to a considerable extent consists of "ancient, obsolete mental mechanisms, generally relegated to the recesses of the psyche where the *primary process* prevails" (Arieti, 1967, p. 328). The primary process in the Freudian system is considered as occurring early in the ontogenetic development, and the secondary type is then gradually substituted as the subject matures. Arieti called the type of thinking supported by primary processes *paleological thinking*; he specifies how logical thinking discriminates on the basis of identity between subjects (A = A and not = B), while paleological thinking discriminates on the identity of attributes (if A and B share a common attribute, then A = B).[4] These primary mechanisms are supposed to reappear in various mental disorders and in the creative process, in which they achieve a special combination with the secondary process mechanism (Arieti calls this combination *"tertiary process"*). The psychotic mind, however, has no mastery over its journey into the unknown and cannot differentiate illusions from different realities nor can it rely on logic to process the emergent material and to anchor it into a healthy sense of what is real.[5]

The emergent thought often surprises the owner because there appears to be a dissimilarity between the analogy and the problem; but it is also accompanied

---

[4] For a schizophrenic mind, if the David of old was connoted with a specific affective cluster and present day John is connoted with the same cluster, then John is certainly David in disguise. Furthermore, if John (or David) loves the guitar, then with all probability everyone else who likes or has a guitar is or is in the same plot as David/John.

[5] I have provided elsewhere (Sanguineti, 1999) detailed examples of these psychotic realities and the affect links supporting them. The affects contained a profound personal truth and therefore colored the delusions with their "reality" attribute.

by a feeling of discovery or recognition (it is recognized, in my opinion, because it has been met before, within the realm of the self); it is unexpected and its inspiration requires a reduction in concentration: "hard work does not pay" (Gelernter, 1994, p. 84). One is reminded of Asimov's (1953/1991) comment, expressed by one of his heroes, Janov Pelorat: "I have found in my own work ... that zeroing tightly on a particular problem is self-defeating. Why not relax... and our unconscious mind ... may solve the problem for us" (p. 109). The "puzzle" that I reported at the beginning of the book is a powerful example of the creative process. It is indeed a true puzzle how those images could emerge from the depths of my "sleeping" brain; images that are more cogent and gravid with transcendent experiential meaning than any one I could produce while in a logical mode of thinking.

In other words, reframing Damasio's comment that the brain knows more than the conscious mind reveals, vast aspects of the domain of the self and its autobiographical memory may continue to remain hidden to the ego. Figure 9-1 schematically identifies the province of the ego, that includes transitional states as the fringe phenomena of William James, "hunches," indefinable feelings, and the like. When seen in this context, the validity of a differentiation of consciousness in the two conditions of ego and self, rather than the core primary and the HOC-extended types, may be better understood. Ego and self represent different dynamics emerging from a sentient brain, the first being primarily an interactional function, gifted with the powerful tool of high-focus logic and adaptively mutating along with the demands of the external world; the latter is a construct that comprises the entire psychic structure; an inner experience that has continuity in time and space. We all have a sense of a stable ego, although probably some of this sense of stability percolates upward out of the self. I invite the reader to reflect on the shifts in ego state when one quickly shifts from being parented to parenting, from professional to social or to lover or to personal[6]: our affective coloration, voice, posture, pattern of thinking change in ways of which we are quite conscious, if we give them attention; but below the interactive layer we are aware of a deep feeling of permanence; we remain also the same self, unless we suffer from a pathology of the self.[7]

A caveat is required at this point: Freud brought the unconscious realm of mind back into psychology; however, he may not have been able to fully shake off the primacy of Cartesian consciousness when he insisted that the ego should phagocyte the self ("where id is, ego shall be") as the corollary for full psychological growth. It is presumed that he referred particularly to those "repressed" areas of the unconscious that contained id states in covert conflict

---

[6] Jung, if I recall correctly, referred to these configurations as personae.

[7] The syndrome of multiple personality disorder, or dissociative identity disorder, is an extreme example of a splintered self pathology.

with healthy conscious adaptation; however, I suspect that the message came to signify that ego consciousness should supervene the entirety of the unconscious aspect of the self. If I am correct then his requirement is like asking that the tip of an iceberg should contain also its base. The ego cannot colonize the self or duplicate it, as this would eventuate in severe overload (as observed in psychotic states); rather, the evolutionary function of the ego consists in applying the available knowledge to the interactive domain and to negotiate the most appropriate survival path; full psychological growth should depend on the development of easy access to the knowledge and reasoning power imbedded in that other state of consciousness, much larger than the ego state, that is called the self.

The evolutionary path seeks the selectional development of easier links between self knowledge and ego knowledge, with a greater integration of the ego state into the structure of the self. Several steps are required to promote such mental evolution and growth; initially there is the need for an expanded acceptance and recognition of the richness and role of unconscious dynamics upon the ego's conscious state; only when this phase is achieved can one begin to focus on how to optimize the channels of communication between the two entities so that the unconscious richness of evolutionary experience can be reliably and knowingly tapped into, and used to negotiate our interactive reality.

To summarize:

- None of the languages appears able or sufficient to resolve the explanatory gap between neural patterns and mental images. Damasio admits that at present the gap cannot be filled; Edelman and Tononi seem to propose that the answer may reside in "more of the same": given a sufficient number of coherent ensembles in the dynamic core then matter will become imagination; however, they do not offer a reasonable explanation of the actual transformation. Furthermore, the flickers of neural patterns, which neuroscience can objectively analyze in many different ways, could never be proven to be the flickers of mental images, even if the recording is simultaneous, because the relationship of these two states (biological and cognitive) remains intrinsically a mystery.

- The first-person language is well fitted to explore the mental side of the gap but could not intrinsically observe the neural patterns to which mental images correlate. The answer to the gap in my opinion cannot be grasped through some mechanism in the domain of the neural science per se, nor could it be grasped through first-person observations from the other side of the canyon; but it might eventually be captured through some "equation" in the domain of nonlinear physics.[8]

---

[8] Equally intriguing is how imagination becomes matter (how mental images—as sounds and written symbols—percolate downward to become neural events and affect other neural events).

- We do not know the dialect of those aspects of the self that are articulated into meaningful dynamics outside the domain of the ego and its conscious mental images; the knowledge of the brain could be coded in purely electrochemical patterns, or already composed in the mysterious code of mental images. We cannot look there, either as objective observers or as subjects. I came to the conclusion that at this level of dynamics the brain deals with nonrepresentational patterns, my VRT; but it is a hunch based on a set of fleeting impressions that I could not really explain. However, all three languages point strongly to the immensity of mind, to the multidimensionality of its dynamics, to the rationale for a vast system of knowledge that could articulate our interaction with the world (internal as well as external; abstract as well as concrete) in ways much more efficient than the slow process we call "logical" or "rational" thinking (what I called RT). All evidence points to the direction of different mental dimensions—for which I have used the common metaphors of self and ego—and to a spectrum of "consciousness" (if we mean by that a state in which rational and meaningful decisions are made, based on "consciousness" of our interactive needs) within which the Cartesian mode resides.

- Finally, the review of these alphabets and their metaphors for mind carries the consistent message that the (human) mind is an absolutely unique phenomenon in each subject: its uniqueness resides in its being the result of chance events (as nonlinear science demonstrates) that have accumulated during the millions of years of each individual's evolutionary and developmental agenda; it finds support in, among others, Edelman's insistence on the nonreplicability and nonlinear computability of the brain; and it has a long history of being recognized as such: Psyche's palace was available to her exclusively, and did not need any guards or locks. And one hopes it will continue to be so, self-protected from objective probes. As a matter of fact I am very concerned by the reflection that if neuroscience could achieve an objective and direct observation of true mental processes—rather than neural patterns whose meanings remain hidden—without the inevitable and obligatory, prerequired mediation of the subject, this achievement would set a condition fraught with the gravest of dangers: the loss of our inner privacy.

In the preceding chapters we have examined different aspects of the psyche as they have been described in the three languages, and found overall a very encouraging concordance on what is described; differences are often due more to semantic preferences than to true discordance; occasionally, superimposing the three models helped to identify the aspects of a model that did not fit the general picture. Figure 9-2 offers an illustration of the main topics discussed above and incorporated into an integrated diagram of mind:

Adaptational data (1) developed during evolution and common to many species (a), to the entire hominid line (b), and to sociocultural organizations

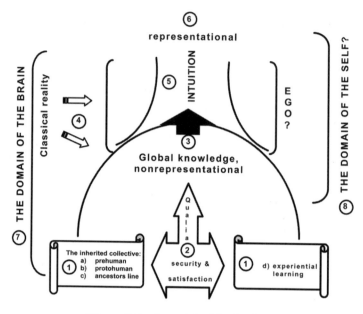

Figure 9-2: A model of (my) mind.

(c) constantly interact with data from the individual's experiential learning
(d) in ways consistent with the findings from evolutionary psychology, with
Edelman's reentry model, with the principles of nonlinear science, and with
mythical literature, starting from the Egyptian description of the "soul."

These data (2) are processed for basic survival value and are in this way
categorized and weighted with qualia (affective loading). This phase reflects
the value-categorization concept of Edelman, the valence-arousal concepts of
Kaszniak, the foundation for the affect-linking process described by Gelernter,
and the overall central role of affectivity in thought production described by
Damasio. It also represents the progressive interaction between Psyche and
Eros, the need for an Eros domain to relate to her and intimately connect with
her.

The data (3) constitute our entire knowledge and are available at an
unconscious, nonrepresentational level in a global and ever-changing way that
is a precursor to conscious awareness. The process operates along nonlinear
parameters in the phase space of the global maps and functional cluster
of Edelman, or Scott's phase space of creativity, or the mythical palace of
Apuleius.

Under activation (4) from classical reality these data eventually give emergence (nonlinear dynamics) to representational constructs (6). The transformation may be perceived as intuition, or insight (5). This is particularly so when
the thought process runs in a low-focus state. The representational constructs,

or mental images, allow for internal as well as external communication and interaction and may involve discrete neuronal networks within the context of a globally activated (binding) state of consciousness. Both nonconscious and conscious conditions are within the domain of the brain (7). The self may be coded in a nonrepresentational as well as a representational mode (8). The ego expresses that sphere of the self that experiences conscious awareness. It includes peripheral phenomena of which the subject is aware but in a vague and indefinite sense, as fringe phenomena and unnamed "feelings."

In closing their book Edelman and Tononi offer a very evocative reflection. They address it to "meaningful sentences in ordinary language or, even better, (of) poetic exchanges..." but I will apply it to all mental phenomena: *"to grasp their meaning requires both the unique phenomenal experience and the historically based culture of each participating individual"* (Edelman & Tononi, 2000, p. 222). Edelman and Tononi point to this uniqueness to support their position as scientists that phenomena having these characteristics are not fit for scientific study "except in some trivial sense" (p. 222). But doesn't the statement represent what mind is truly about?

PART III

Applying the Knowledge

Chapter 10

THE THREE LANGUAGES AND SCIENCE: A NEW SCIENTIFIC PARADIGM?

The question was: Does Edelman and Tononi's statement represent what mind is truly about? My answer is that it certainly does so. Any science of the human mind that does not accept the uniqueness of such a mind as its fundamental premise is a science without a real subject for study. Philosopher John Searle (1992) emphasized that if a science is not able to explain an aspect of the universe, what should be changed is the science, not the universe. The differences between minds are incredibly greater than the structural similarities and the patterns of neuronal functioning of those brains. Actually, even at the structural level the differences are impressive, as Edelman points out. It follows that the objective language of neuroscience is invaluable in describing stochastic ensembles and in illustrating a certain and generalizable modus operandi of neural patterns up to a level of tremendous complexity as the dynamic core. However, this approach has to fall short of what concerns the mental dimension itself; the dimension of personal meanings and purposes to which the brain is eventually geared. This is a field that cannot be explored and understood without giving primary attention to its individuality: any understanding of self consciousness, as a dynamic phenomenon or process of negotiating the act of living in a meaningful and private way, requires an understanding of the self. We cannot appreciate how mind operates without exploring these operations through the knowledge of what are the unique characteristics that dictate the mental outcomes. By this I mean that even the neural patterns, while stochastically "similar," will very likely prove to be profoundly different when applied to the real subject. Scientific knowledge is now often simply equated with objective knowledge and it is requested to be observer independent; as we have discussed, these are two egregious limitations that exclude the study of subjective phenomena. Professor Morton Reiser (2001) states that mental and brain sciences, pertaining to two different domains, use different languages; their concepts are framed at different levels of abstraction.[1] A great deal of the sterility of academic psychology over the last 50 years has come from a persistent failure to recognize and come to terms with the fact that the ontology of the mental is an irreducibly first-person ontology. Human consciousness is a mental phenomenon that requires matter to become imagination, and imagination is subjectivity.

The problem with the two domains and their respective languages is not an insignificant one. Let us consider a simple instance: the mechanism involved in the mental image of a pure sensation, a *traditional* quale, observed from the objective perspective. The first difficulty that we encounter is that pure sensations (primary unadulterated neural patterns) probably are never available to experimental research. No sensory experience can be organized as a neural pattern (not to speak of a mental pattern) without being immediately modified: a specific band of radiation for a primary color (say yellow) is undoubtedly the same to every retinal field; once translated into an electrochemical neural pattern it inevitably becomes "impure," already in its first relay station, the lateral geniculate, through reentrant connections. By the time it reaches its specific cortical stations it will have been recorded, compared, recognized and categorized, survival-assessed, qualia-weighted, recategorized, stabilized in a comprehensive neural pattern, and eventually translated into a mental pattern and percolated upward into HOC to become a truly conscious sensory experience. That specific electrochemical pattern does not need to reach the primary visual cortex in order to be recognized by the brain for what it means and to be complemented with a quale definition.

The second difficulty is that even if one gives up the idea of "purity" and accepts the conglomerate as the expression of the "yellow quale" (Edelman has upgraded his quale definition to this level), the neural pattern could be traced objectively, but could not be invested with a meaning unless the perceiving subject gives a report (verbal or behavioral, from ego consciousness or unknowingly). Only when correlated with the subjective experience of a sensation would the specific neural noise under observation—one among all the neural background activities going on simultaneously—receive confirmation that it indeed reflects the stimulus.

A third, and formidable difficulty has to deal with recognizing due process to mental events and the happenstance of connective dynamics. The primary pathways for the sensory experience are certainly well established and their

---

[1] "Top-down data from psychoanalytic and related clinical psychological studies should be evaluated and taken into account with data from the bottom-up neurobiologic sciences. Psychological sciences gain access to unique, often hidden, personal aspects of human experience that are not accessible to biologic methods of investigation. Surely it is reasonable to expect this kind of information to supplement and complement, rather than conflict with, neurobiologic information."

neural dynamics could be followed—at least in theory—with sufficient reliability despite the variations within the system related to its epigenetic unfolding. Always in theory, one could trace the receptive-expressive loop—the primary neural mechanics of sensory input and motor response. But these objective readings would be profoundly inadequate unless the affective component is identified too; and here is where major trouble begins, because this component is absolutely idiosyncratic and unique to the subject. And yet, this affect link is the component that specifies mind: let me repeat here Gelernter's position: "The first step in a computer model of mind ought to be a computer model of the cognitive spectrum. If we don't know how to build such a model, we have no idea how a truly convincing fake mind would actually work" (p. 43). No fake model of mind could be convincing unless it integrates affective resonance in a very fundamental way; it follows that no comprehensive model can achieve such integration unless it undertakes the painstaking task of tracing the affectivity package[2] within which one could eventually identify the conscious and unconscious affects linked to the sensory experience for that specific mind. Consider my apple web as I lay in the reclining surgical chair (Sanguineti, 1999, p. 3). The mask of the controlled image releaser (CIR) is set with a tight seal over my face and I stare into the dense gray fog that fills the mask and my entire visual field. At carefully calculated intervals the image of a ripe, red apple flashes rapidly in the center of the field. Nearby, the neurosurgical team observes on a monitor the patterns of graded colored concentrations painted on my brain by the precisely titrated sequential infusions of radio-labeled chemicals. The apple appearances illuminate a bright and stable web of interconnected pathways, easily recognizable among the variegated and unstable permutations of diffuse colors that reflect the distribution of each wave of radioisotopes. The composite computerized image of the web becomes clearer with each successive stimulus and its definition increases (as a shallow reef would do by breaking the progression of the waves to the shore). This three-dimensional web traces the "apple-perceiving" phenomena from the retinal cells of my eyes to the "recognition" centers in my occipital lobe. It also includes the predicted branch to the labeling site in my brain. In a nearby surgical recliner you undergo the same procedure: you too are repeatedly presented with an identical image of a red apple as precisely positioned as mine is. The computer now superimposes our two webs on the upper half of each screen, while continuously upgrading the images as more information is added with each new exposure. Predictably, the two images are remarkably

---

[2] This package will also consist of neural patterns in the brain; when one looks "from the outside" at this complex dance it might be quite difficult to actually specify which dancer does which movement.

similar and allow for a very gratifying level of matching. Only minor blurs, well within acceptable variance, interrupt the clarity of the juxtaposed design.

The neurosurgical transplant team, satisfied with the high compatibility of the two images, applies the probes of the electrochemical transplanter (ECT) to a preformed window in my skull. With astounding precision the probes gradually recognize and dissect the apple web along its electrochemical boundaries with the rest of my neural tissue. Microchemical and electrical markers are left at each synaptic stump site for future recognition. As the process unfolds, the dissected part of the web is constantly surrounded by the feeding broth that keeps it alive and protects its architecture in space from any disruptive mechanical stress.

At the nearby recliner your apple web is equally dissected away. Once the dissections are completed, the broth-filled containers slide on their tracks from one recliner to the other. The ECT mode is reversed, and each transplanter begins the delicate and precise process of identifying each marker and rebuilding the electrochemical bonds between the transplanted parts and the rest of the organ. Minute adjustments (the blurs in the juxtaposed pictures) are gently smoothed over through the plasticity of the surrounding tissues. The two-way transplant is now complete. I recognize with absolute ease the red apple that flashes inside my CIR, and so do you.

What you and I have been subjected to is a transplant of the "stimulus perception and recognition" neural circuitry in our brain. This circuitry transmits the attributes of external reality deep into the brain, in a very predictable way. The process is a significant aspect of consciousness (as well as nonconscious automatic monitoring of external reality). *But it is not the subjective experience.*

Now consider the "yellow quale" of Edelman; its processing into a conscious state becomes immediately related to earlier experiences with that specific color. Imagine that previous and affectively loaded exposures to the color yellow made it strongly "unpleasant." As for the immune system, the "antigen" represented by the electrochemical pattern of yellow will be immediately recognized and tagged with a negative valence. By the time the sequence reaches consciousness it is already a complex sensation spread along a time continuum. By that time, its predominant valence will also have reverberated along multiple affective links coded with the same emotional palette, for further, more elaborate discrimination. Value systems will by now have been involved, spreading the process to multiple levels of assemblies, or "maps." The connectivity of the mental pattern supporting the mental image will be quite complex and it may be quite different from the pattern of another "yellow" in another mind. It is likely that, if we could capture the two "yellow" networks in their entirety, they would look quite dissimilar.

The case of JD offers strong support to the visual "yellow quale" scenario, but in another sensory modality. Bright, well educated and witty, JD, now in her late thirties, suffered from recurrent depression but primarily she suffered from truly malignant alcoholism that had resisted multiple treatment attempts and programs. During the first 2 years of therapy several trials at abstinence had all been short-lived while she continued to present the specter and active fantasy of suicide. The exploration of her addictive relationship to alcohol had evidenced a true love affair with the chemical, and in this way she differed somewhat from many chronic alcoholics who intermittently verbalize despair and hatred for the control that alcohol visibly has on their entire life. She loved the taste of alcohol, she loved the way it made her feel ("warm and cozy and safe") and she particularly loved its smell; bringing a glass of alcohol to her nostrils and inhaling its "scent" was a quasi-religious experience (she would never drink beer because to her it smelled bad).

She was an only child. Her parents, affluent and old money with roots in the 13 colonies, were described as cold, unemotional WASPS, who lived dysfunctional lives behind the facade of social respectability and were "functional alcoholics" themselves. She recounted often how her mother would never hold her or kiss her; when mother did so out of social expectations or obligation, she would experience her mother's embrace as physically cold and tense, awkward. This had been particularly true since she had been 5 or 6 years old. She had also, though, a set of earlier memories of her mother occasionally picking her up in an embrace that would be different: the embrace would then feel warm and supple; the mother's very skin would be the source of such warmth.

During one particular session, as she was again recalling such embraces with the memories of a 3-year-old, she mentioned: "I seem to remember now that she smelled different, in those moments; I would tell her 'you smell good' and she would laugh." Here she paused, and then continued: "Her breath smelled different; it smelled of... sure! She smelled of alcohol! That is why she was so fuzzy and affectionate on those occasions."

That was the extra and unrelenting power of the chemical: the "pure" olfactory sensation of the little child was also the memory of a smell, the kinesthetic memory of a "good" embrace warmed up and disinhibited by alcohol, the memory of a loving mother. It is worth noting that within months after this affect link came into ego consciousness and its meanings were processed, the addiction began to assume an increasingly sour taste, new values took the place of old ones, meta-stable synaptic systems got reconfigured, old attractors moved in the background and new ones began to take their place, and after few more months she achieved her first prolonged period of abstinence, on her way to sobriety.[3]

---

[3] I invite the reader to explore at this point the "qualia complex" that has become activated by the description of the case, to try and identify if its overall valence is favorable or unfavorable, and to reflect if and how the balance affects the reader's *scientific attitude* toward

How can this complexity be studied? How can we explore the subjectivity of "yellow," which is a much closer representation of the human mind than its neural patterns without a meaning? When neuroscientific experiments replicate and trace stochastically sensory pathways via sophisticated radioimaging techniques or elaborated virtual models, what happens of these profound differences? Where do they hide? How could they be included in the scientific equation? How can a neuroscience be devised that would simultaneously utilize the two levels of description of the biological and of the cognitive hierarchy, and use the two languages in a truly complementary way? I do not know how it could be done. Maybe it cannot be done. Maybe, as mentioned earlier, it cannot be done because of the constraints of scientific materialism, in which case we need to seriously seek another scientific paradigm for neurosciences. Scott had pointed out that the paradigm for the science of the 19th and 20th centuries had been the Machine and that the science of the 21st century should look elsewhere for a new model, and he suggested that the Poem could be such a model. When I heard him I thought he was formulating a nice poetic metaphor until I realized that he was actually describing science.

The pervading philosophy of the machine is expressed to an extreme by psychoanalyst Donna Haraway (1991). She takes a position that addresses the enlistment of the machine as an intrinsic part of our culture. In doing this she provides a fitting example of Gelernter's concern about our relationship to the machine and the danger from excessive reliance on, and identification with it. She challenges the traditional dependence on the organic and essentialist models of humanity; she underlines how all attempts to separate us from other living organisms have failed, and concurrently the inherent humanity of those specific attributes as autonomy, free will, and creativity, that were supposed to separate us from the machine, is also becoming challenged and less exclusive. Humanity is therefore poised between a lost myth of nature and a futuristic dream of perpetual technological revolution. Psychologically, she labels such standing as being a cyborg, part cybernetic machine and part living organism. The cyborg may represent the ultimate expression of linear, computational processing and the concept is not as futuristic as it might seem. Human robotics (the use of mechanical devices to replace defective human parts) is becoming a well accepted and strongly supported endeavor, the interface between the computer and the human is constantly sliced down, made "consumer friendly"; the idea of downloading directly from the Web into our brain modules for happiness or pleasure or excitation is most likely already under study; virtual reality games, in which the brain is tricked into experiencing nonexisting situations as real, are just the startups of a new market.

---

the material presented. This introspective assessment of affective valences is a routine aspect of psychotherapy, dictated by the need to maintain the observer's neutrality.

As I mentioned earlier, Scott's proposal of the poem as a new scientific metaphor is actually quite consistent with the nonlinearity characteristic to the biological world in its comparison of the dynamics of mind to the dynamics of a poem. The emergence of a poem is a very good example of the workings of the brain along nonlinear and emergentist directions, where the dynamics grasp and elaborate a specific theme within the phase space of creativity. The visible outcome is quite different from the sum of its parts.

Edelman and Tononi illustrate fittingly their concerns and constraints concerning the inclusion of "poetic utterances" into the field of neuroscientific research by reporting part of a poem (CXXVI) by Emily Dickinson (1830–1886):

> The brain — is wider than the sky —
> for — put them side by side —
> The one the other will contain
> With ease — and You — beside — (ca. 1862)

We cannot ultimately escape the fact that the true workings of the mind are represented in the four lines above. When Edelman and Tononi chose the phrase "where matter becomes imagination" as the subtitle for their book, they chose the poem as the final quest in searching for a solution to the process of transformation. It seems therefore appropriate to briefly examine Dickinson's statement through the prism of the three languages. Several points are worth commenting on.

First, the content is truly impressive. Behind the facade, which evokes a predominantly poetic metaphor, a deeper level of intuitive knowledge percolates upward. I do not know to what extent Dickinson was familiar with the neural anatomy and neurophysiology of the 19th century. Electrophysiology was very rudimentary at best; the voices of Sherrington, Freud, and James were still to be heard of. Yet, she decided to focus her attention on the brain (not on the mind) and in these four lines she captured its hyperimmense quality as poignantly as the three scientific models on which this book is organized. Her statement that the brain contains the sky and the self correlates very well with the data from neuroscience and its mathematics as they have been presented earlier on: the number of possible neural circuits range in the realm of 10 followed by at least a million zeros, while there are only a puny 10 followed by 79 zeros, give or take a few, particles of matter in the entire universe. The brain can indeed contain the sky with a lot to spare.[4]

---

[4] The present book was well into its printing process when I read Dr. Edelman's last work (Edelman, 2004). Although described as a review of his research for the general reader, the book—aptly titled *Wider Than the Sky* in reference to Dickinson's poem—implies novel perspectives, not found in his previous writings. They elaborate and realign crucial issues, even

The form in which the poem conveys such knowledge raises interesting responses; at one level it is more or less "touching," depending on one's poetic inclinations; at another level it may "ring" true, such ringing being based on the reader's affective resonance;[5] at yet another level, the one of traditional neuroscience, it is often considered unfit to be a scientific subject ("It is enough to recognize that some scientifically founded objects are not appropriate scientific subjects"; Edelman &· Tononi, 2000, p. 222). In my opinion, the intuitive knowledge of the brain's immensity evident in Dickinson's work should represent an essential subject of scientific research rather than being dismissed as "unproven" or a beautiful mystical utterance. Such examples of logically unexplainable knowledge contain profound, fundamental information

---

more closely than before, to some of the views expounded in this book. There are several instances of these "novelties"—and of some softening in the "objective observer" stance that rigidly guided all his previous works. Like his admission, while discussing consciousness (C) and its neural substrate (C^l), that the subjective position is crucial in experiencing and studying consciousness: "given that it is a property entailed by C^l, C is the only information on C^l available to a subject" (p. 116); or like the importance of value systems in the very formation of conscious states: "from a causal point of view, the reverse is also true—only as a result of value systems in a selectional brain can the bases emerge for the phenomenal gift of consciousness." (p. 139) (I refer the reader to my definition of brain formulated on p. 56, footnote #13); or like his addressing the difference between (Cartesian) logic and analogical thinking as they relate to creativity (pp. 147–148). To my knowledge this is the first time that Edelman openly addresses the themes expounded in detail in Chapters 8 and 9 of this book. He seems to consider the selectional, "degenerate" workings of the core (C^l) as the site for analogical abilities ("selectional thinking"), that counterpoint the logical mode of thinking; he fundamentally aligns himself to the position that I share with Gelernter when he states that "while logic can prove theorems ... it cannot choose axioms." And again: "the products of metaphorical abilities, while necessarily ambiguous, can be richly creative. Logic is not creative but it can tame the excesses of creative pattern thinking." (p. xx) This is clearly analogous to the pattern of low focus thinking described on p. 85 and again on p. 94 of this book. He concludes the discussion with an interesting metaphor: "selectionism is the mistress of our thoughts, while logic is their housekeeper." (p. xx) By substituting "Muse" to "mistress" one would have "The Muse in the Machine" metaphor of Gelernter. By substituting "Eros" one would have Apuleius' myth.

Finally: at the conclusion of his book *A Universe of Consciousness* Dr. Edelman presented the poem as an utterance unfit for scientific investigation, and he appeared firm in his position that subjective data are also not appropriate for consciousness research. Yet in this last work he identifies consciousness with the same poem, having been captured by the same mystery that captured my attention: the poet's metaphorical—but quite accurate!—description of the human brain. "I find it impressive that, in extolling the width and depth of the mind, Dickinson referred exclusively to the brain." (p. XIII) In addition, his conclusions offer a striking example of the message contained in *The Rosetta Stone*: the invaluable use of the three languages and how they enrich our understanding of the mental universe. Perhaps, Dr. Edelman's next work will start with the mistress (or Muse) metaphor, to explore how housekeeper and mistress (Psyche and Eros) need equal representation and cooperative feedback in order to assure the fullest expression of a human's mind.

[5] Gelernter (1994) has a lot to say about poetic language in the last section of his book.

about (1) the dynamics of the brain; (2) what do the libraries consist of; and (3) how they are transmitted, stored, and activated. Our ability to put together a decent model of mind would be rather slim, unless we come to some understanding of how the brain comes up with such dazzling performances; because this is the habitual way in which the brain works, from the Egyptian Sekhem and Ba to Psyche and to Dickinson; and to us.

A second comment relates to the organization of the processes that eventuate in the emergence of the poem. The creative act is a unique phenomenon (the violinist Paganini was insistent on his own unreplicability!); nevertheless it is also a common one if we include its garden varieties that color our daily lives. Its dynamics are better represented, and analyzable, in a poem than in a reductive situation directed by the objective scenario of the experimental laboratory. This scenario is extremely useful, of course, and indeed invaluable in exploring complex neural patterns; but the mental pattern requires an approach that would allow for the inclusion and consideration of the entire set of dimensions that define its phase space. The ability of the brain to condense immense meanings into a very economic—24 words!—and yet very realistic final outcome is a stunning one.

The organization of the logical discourse is guided by the selectional workings of affectivity. An emotional package orchestrates the connectivity web out of which the semantic choices emerge under supervision by the ego. The package is quite complex: it includes diverse aspects of the affectivity dimensions, from qualia to values, to specific emotions, and to feelings linking the present to past memories; the phase space is constellated with multiple "established" attractors, most of which are common to humanity but whose combination and order of priority are subtly unique to each mind. The semantic choices are selected specifically to convey both a verbal representation of the creative product and an affective one: a true marriage of Psyche and Eros. The emotional package that is so masterfully conveyed—much of it being undefined and possibly operating mainly in the unconscious—has to have a pivotal role in the touching and deeply relational power of these 24 words. Here we can perhaps intersubjectively assess the affect link and start to develop a better grasp on what Damasio (1999) calls the nonverbal vocabulary of feelings.

My point is that the human mind *is this subjectivity within the brain*. Damasio recognizes, more than Edelman and Tononi do, its intrinsic scientific value and the necessity of it being included in the sciences of the mind, although the last two authors concur by concluding that the key to the world knot lies in the poem. To untangle the knot will truly open the dimension of mental images to scientific exploration, and therefore "psychological" neuroscientists have to stop lateralizing the brain to the level where it is a necessary but non significant piece of matter; while "biological" neuroscientists have to do likewise with subjectivity, rather than stunt any interest in its study by declaring it an unfit scientific object. Rather, a reformulated neuroscience has to learn how to concurrently operate in the two languages of the two domains. Perhaps, we all have to revisit our territoriality and dominance programs and the affects out of which our sense of truth emerges.

By chance, I had found in some now forgotten science-fiction book the following anonymous poem (or fragment of a poem):

> I hide my wings inside my soul
> Their feathers soft and dry
> And when the world's not looking
> I take them out and fly.

I had kept it as a scrap of paper on my desk where, defying annihilation, it got shuffled from one pile to the next for over 2 years. Its mention of a soul had naturally intrigued me, and I had briefly reflected that it was a nice metaphor for the psychotherapeutic process and the privacy of mind.

Its final resurfacing happened while I had become interested in the first verse of the Dickinson poem quoted by Edelman and Tononi; I saw it as balancing nicely the brain description with a mind description. This second poem too is a remarkable example of an economic emergentism of a state of mind from a phase space whose dimensions we could only very faintly and inadequately "feel."

Only much later, puzzled by this felt symmetry, I looked at it more closely and realized that it contained 24 words. Due to my serendipitous connection of one poem to the other, the fact that these two pieces of creative work about brain and mind would be so strangely duplicative was an oddity that I found difficult to digest as such. I thought that perhaps Dickinson had written the second poem too, although its quality did not match up; but when I reviewed her entire work I could not find it anywhere. If they are indeed the product of two different minds striving to capture the same "object," couldn't the symmetry in content themes (sky, inside, and outside) and semantic economy point to some "rule" or common process—not limited only to the constraints of poetic requirements— that directs the brain in creating images?

If we can agree on the fact that the information emerging through a creative act is material fit for scientific research, then when a human mind communicates a script about a mental process (i.e., transfers into symbols what is happening within its cognitive hierarchy) the neuroscientist ought to examine the products very carefully and exhaustingly. They represent the best, if not the only data available about those types of processes; it is like looking directly into the vials and glass tubes and other paraphernalia of a chemical experiment. The demotic language of the psychological domain offers the most complete translation of the mental apparatus presently available. However, its appropriate use to conduct neuroscientific research and to understand mental phenomena requires an appreciation and attention to its consistency with its neurobiological counterpart; otherwise it could be marred by vagueness and lack of foundations. The observer language of the neurobiological domain is indispensable to grasping the underlying electrochemistry, and someday it may contribute to an understanding of the explanatory gap; however, this language may run the risk of some degree of artificiality if it avoids the natural complex workings of the mind as its subject, and limits its own symbolism to the contracted and bound sets of data that fit the experimental bench of the psychological laboratory or the artificial design of a virtual "brain"—and "mind."

The language and framework of scientific materialism has proven unfit to explain mind, and, therefore, in accordance with the suggestion by Searle reported at the beginning of this chapter, the science has to be changed; nonlinear science offers a realistic and functional alternative to linearity, and its fundamental concepts should come to guide all our experimentations and speculations. The nonlinear framework does indeed allow a sufficient latitude to begin and perceive, in some indistinct way, how the brain creates images, and images that are always unique. The formulation and application of both first-person and third-person languages to the study of mind, and in my opinion to the clinical arena as well, need to reflect, and be consistent with, the ideographic language of the set of rules that define all biological phenomena. If such "translation" is muddled or forced then something is "fishy" concerning the psychological or the biological metaphors.

To conclude, and to repeat myself yet another time, I will paraphrase Jung's (1958) example of a bed of pebbles (p. 16), that he used to critique certain aspects of the statistical method in the study of the human mind:

1. Scientific materialism is very efficient in measuring the mean characteristics (as weight or volume) of a stable and replicable sample, or a sample that has been stabilized by dismissing any implicit irregularity, as a bed of pebbles or a human cohort.
2. In the biological world, and specifically in the case of mind, irregularity is the predominant characteristic; understanding mind requires understanding the specific attributes of each single pebble—understanding the differences.
3. The statistical mean values provided by scientific materialism may never be found in any of the individual pebbles.
4. A comprehensive science of mind will therefore include the analysis of neuronal ensembles and neural patterns together with the analysis of mental events; that is, of subjectivity.[6]

---

[6] Damasio (1999): "Subjective entities require, as do objective ones, that enough observers undertake rigorous observations according to the same experimental design; ... knowledge gathered from subjective observation, e.g., introspective insights, can inspire objective ex-

5. Such science will by necessity have to operate along principles different from the linear ones.

6. The science will require the study of the conscious/unconscious matrix (the psychological self, the neural dynamic core) that contains the libraries of knowledge, side by side with the study of ego consciousness—or the state that verifies the fit between knowledge and the demands of reality.

---

periments, and, no less importantly, subjective experiences can be explained in terms of the available scientific knowledge. The idea that the nature of subjective experiences can be grasped effectively by the study of their behavioral correlates is wrong" [p. 309].

Chapter 11

THE THREE LANGUAGES AND TREATMENT

If the different languages and dimensions are crucial to the formulation of a more integrated neuroscience, they are even more so in the clinical field, where the guiding parameters that will determine specific outcomes will affect in profoundly subjective ways the life of a real, and suffering, human psyche. When the treatment of a wounded mind is entertained, innumerable dimensions are at stake: from coping mechanisms addressing the psychic and physical pain to overall adaptive behaviors encompassing the larger landscape of persons and events surrounding the painful situation; from the effect of the wound upon the relatedness toward others and the world to the very emotional palette of the experience of living (the feeling of what happens). The wound may originate from a structural, anatomical injury or from a psychological one, but eventually it becomes the subjective experience of the wound itself, an experience that ultimately affects all areas of a person's life. In this situation, the knowledge and the perspective that can be acquired by the trilingual translation of the condition and of its plan for treatment achieve their clearest resolution and prove to be the most beneficial.

In an admittedly very simplified form, the two currently favored models of psychopathology either view the disorders of the mind to be related to primary (inherited or epigenetic) errors in neurotransmission ("a disease of the synapses") that eventuate in disturbances of thoughts, affects, and behavior; or consider them to be related to internalized memories of past experiences (affective as well as cognitive) that cascade downward and may produce disturbances in patterns of neurotransmission as collateral effects.

Figure 11-1 encapsulates a view of treatment that respects and incorporates the three domains; its main points will be exemplified in the course of the next two chapters by clinical vignettes.

The diagram of the cognitive hierarchy occupies the center of Figure 11-1, which illustrates how the neurobiologic and the psychotherapeutic approaches relate to the hierarchy, at which level they are most likely to exert their initial

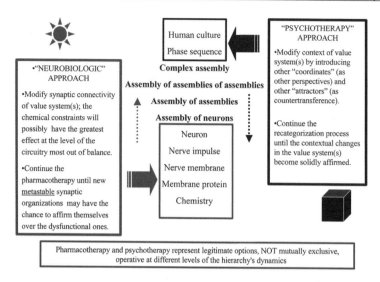

Figure 11-1: A trilingual perspective of treatment.

effect, and the causal direction of their constraints upon other levels of the hierarchy.

The present state of research on the physiopathology of "mental disorders," or psychiatric syndromes, irrespective of the etiology, is articulated around disturbances in neurotransmission and conceptualizes treatment as providing some degree of interference and manipulation of the main monoaminergic systems as the dopaminergic, serotonergic, and noradrenergic. These complexes reflect: the value systems of Edelman and Tononi; the affective valence and role of feelings of Damasio, Kaszniak, Gelernter, and Apuleius; and they can be visualized as stable and powerful attractors in the phase space of mind schematized in Figure 2-3.

The therapeutic process can therefore include:

1. An effort toward diffuse manipulation of specific neural systems by the use of agents that interact with the neurotransmission of those systems and consequently might dampen dysphoric affectivity or obligated behavior. Such a modality of treatment is outlined in the left box of Figure 11-1 (the large arrows indicate the levels of the hierarchy that are primarily affected by each type of intervention). The upper-directed gray arrow suggests the direction of causality toward upper levels. This approach has proven to be rather successful. It will not change any contextual issue that might be present, because a change in meanings and values requires the use of mental images and a dialogue (internal as well as external) with ego participation; but it could be presumed that the ongoing modification of specific assemblies will preferentially facilitate new synaptic webs and neurally induce a change in the meaning of the mental

image. The time needed to maintain such dampening in order to achieve permanent change is a great unknown, given the innumerable variables pulling different weights to the process.

2. An attempt to modify the contextual issue by exploring and addressing the higher levels of the hierarchy and by constructing a reframed cognitive and affective version of the values and meanings that through their emotional links are driving the distorted experience of the situation. This project calls for the manipulation of events and feelings. Such manipulation requires that the subject begins by revisiting isolated experiences, using his or her specific emotional and cognitive language; these experiences can then be connected into patterns that will illuminate the central systems of meanings and values that put constraints upon the outcome; the subject can then begin to recategorize and reframe their affective valence and to develop a more adaptive emotional package and perception of reality.

Figure 11-2 connects back to the example presented in Figure 2-3 and suggests a very schematic model that reflects what we have seen about nonlinear brain function. An exaggerated values system (serotonergic, dopaminergic, noradrenergic, cholinergic, histaminergic), reflecting an enduring emotional package, has a downward effect upon specific assemblies of neurons.

Whenever these assemblies are recruited in response to certain environmental stimuli or conditions, they exercise downward constraints (at the level of the neuronal membrane and impulse transmission, by altering neuromodulators, etc.) upon neural patterns and therefore incite the obligated, recurrent symptom complex. This symptoms complex (obsessions, compulsions, depressed mood) feeds recursively the exaggerated value system and the loop may eventuate in an endless repetition of an explicit mental pattern (a thought, a behavior, an affect).

The overall survival weight of the attractor—how large it looms within that specific mind—will specify the intermittent or chronic character of the symptomatic outcome and its degree of severity.

When the clinical situation reflects the schema depicted in Figure 11-1, then clearly the combined approach offers the best chance for a satisfactory outcome. KG is a middle-aged woman with a degree in chemistry who works at a basic research center. She has been diagnosed as a paranoid schizophrenic since her midtwenties. She has a wonderful sense of humor and a warm and heartfelt laughter; she is also convinced that after she falls asleep she can become a quite perverse sadomasochistic sexual predator, maybe even a murderer, although her "victims" may actually seek her interest and eagerly "invite" her ministrations. She has never remembered a single shred of evidence from such activity (actually, in her waking state she is a very inhibited and shy individual, with very low self-esteem, describing herself as genitally immature), nor has anyone at any time explicitly accused her or reported her

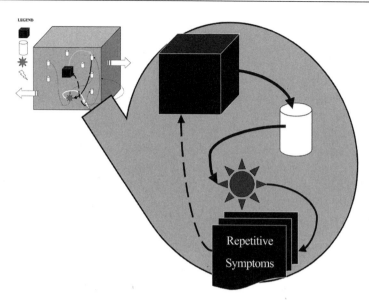

Figure 11-2: A pathological attractor system and its constraint upon symptom formation.

to the authorities. Nevertheless, she is fully convinced that a network of people across the entire country, and possibly abroad as well, know of her activities and inform her episodically, by coughing discreetly when they are around her, that her behavior is a known fact and that she is under surveillance.

KC reported a significant reduction of her intense distress, her despair, and the frightening auditory hallucinatory experiences since she became stabilized on a particular antipsychotic, and she has taken the chemical religiously for several years. Her delusional belief, however, has remained untouched despite several years of "supportive," "educational" psychotherapy. She interprets her entire social environment as adversarial and judgmental, and innocuous comments quite often become colored with denigratory innuendos. As a consequence she has lived a crippled and isolated life, rich in pain and self-doubts.

Once she started the present trial of therapy the contrast between the two configurations became quickly evident: the diurnal shy and self-debasing Ms. Jekyll contrasting the fantasy of the nocturnal all-powerful, sexually exploitative Ms. Hyde. Working on the premise that Ms. Hyde was a delusion of restitution[1] against the reality of Ms. Jekyll—a process that had grown out

---

[1] A delusion of restitution is a psychotic construct that allows the subject to correct an otherwise depriving reality and an unfulfilled drive, and to provide or restore a certain degree of security and satisfaction. It also restitutes a meaning (albeit psychotic) to the otherwise perplexing and unexplainable change in internal and external reality.

of control into a frightening amplification of early, more subdued fantasies of sexual grandeur—the therapy centered cautiously on the negative value system that she had carried in her since early adolescence and that had found confirmation in the progressively increasing "oddity" of her relationships with her social system. Her oddities had caused either puzzlement or openly demeaning, hurtful feedback from others (rather than the normal consensual validation upon which the subject gradually stabilizes its self and ego representations), which had furthered her self-doubts. Once her trust in the therapist appeared to be well established, and with the help of her unusual capacity for self-directed humor, this hypertrophic negative and paranoid value system was recategorized over and over against her achievements, and the discordance between her subjective reality and the intersubjective reality of the therapist was repeatedly revisited. Gradually—oh, so gradually!—the attractor appeared to recede somewhat from the center of her internal landscape: the intensity of the belief showed some fault lines; the distortions of reality became less automatic and more easily challenged; self-reflection and self-constraints against the automatic paranoid interpretations helped her to create a buffer zone between her ego and the archaic affect-driven products of her personal schizophrenic reality. Attempts at socialization became less frightening as she could entertain the possibility that occasional but inevitable rejections could be "normal" rather than invested with a personal paranoid significance. These interventions could not have been possible if specific neural patterns had not been dampened down by the "antipsychotic" agent; only then could the value systems, which had been organized out of an ongoing dysfunctional evaluation of reality, be gradually challenged without simply exacerbating the syndrome and carrying the therapist too into the paranoid world of the psychosis.

This conceptualization of treatment illustrated in Figure 11-1 fosters a continuous awareness of the system of hierarchies and of the recursive influences among multiple levels of dynamics; it also allows a glimpse into the complexity of mental activity. In this way it protects from the risk of putting excessive emphasis on one specific methodology or speculating simplistic modules by reducing the mental structure to just one or a selected few components. Some considerations come to mind that are quite relevant to what I am now discussing. As a starter, we need to agree that the chemical modulation of an affective entity such as a "depression" actually, for all we know, affects a complex cascade of values and feeling states among which the complex syndrome we label with the metaphor of depression covers only a certain spectrum (we really know very little about the intrinsic characteristics of what we call depression).[2] Other affective states not necessarily dysfunctional

---

[2] "Depression" and "anxiety" have been systematically separated in the official psychiatric classification of mental disorders. Recent trends support with growing confidence a "spectrum

will be affected, but the pharmacotherapist may be inattentive to these states because they are not recognized to begin with or, if recognized, are given no consideration unless their changes eventuate in symptoms and behavioral problems. All listed side-effects quoted in the pharmaceutical pamphlets are effects that have reached clinical significance; collateral effects that do not reach such a threshold are not even perceived, although they might change the emotional palette of the person's life, and not only for the better.

When we consider the vast connectivity of a monoaminergic value system we come to understand how by putting constraints on its neuromodulatory functions, and therefore manipulating its hypothetical state of abnormal re-activity, we could indeed counteract some phenomenological distress related to the system's dynamics, but the effect would be widespread and include all sorts of undetectable outcomes. We would achieve a chemically constrained phase space (we would not address the true movement of the heart and the standing of that mind in relation to the world); a space that in the process often becomes creatively diminished from its normal potential. Persons gifted with the emotional acuity mentioned by Gelernter frequently comment that they feel emotionally stunted, or muted, by the chemical intervention; some prefer the pain of the clinical syndrome to the loss of affective resonance. If the psychopharmacologist operates mainly in a high-focus condition and listens to the report of a low-focus mind, he or she may not comprehend such subjective report or discard it as "the lesser of two problems." If the case involves someone such as TP (p. 88) in whom emotions were massively repressed, then any change in the affective spectrum would go unnoticed but for the lessening of the "heaviness" that constituted the conscious perception of his depressive state as this state reached clinical threshold. In other words, when we provoke a pharmacological mutation we need to keep in mind the intricacy of the neural phase space as it was reported in Chapter 2.

Conversely, there is also a great risk in a psychotherapy that: (1) deals essentially with the here and now without exploring and addressing the intricate feedback loops that might be operative among upper and lower levels of the cognitive hierarchy, connecting past experiential memories with current ones; (2) does not consider and identify the presence of any basic abnormality in a major neural circuitry, which would promote abnormal neural patterns and interfere with the recategorization of value-related information; (3) attributes a vast array of psychological distress to one "primary" causative factor (as the Freudian sexual triangle), while ignoring others. Such a one-dimensional

---

model" of illness in which these states are not as sharply differentiated as the DSM lists convey, but, rather, are intertwined in complex ways. The pharmaceutical companies quickly picked up on the idea and the old "exclusive" antidepressants are now repackaged and reformulated as also effective for anxiety.

approach may act as a temporary pacifier—the same way as a chemical could—but it fails to heal or to provide a durable amelioration of the syndrome by promoting enduring changes into self organization and into ego consciousness.

I have given greater critical attention to the risk from excessive reliance on the chemistry of the brain, because of the profoundly dangerous and limiting messages that recently have emerged from the science of psychopharmacology. These messages promulgate the exclusive healing power of psychoactive agents and have openly devalued and discounted the field of the psychotherapies, impervious to the vast accumulation of seminal data on the extraordinarily complex organization of psyche that have emerged from psychological science. In his excellent review of the interaction between neuroscience and the economic objectives of the pharmaceutical companies, Elliott Valenstein (1998) writes: "various support groups, often funded by large grants from the pharmaceutical industry, exaggerate and sometimes distort the effectiveness of drug treatment and what is known about the relationship of brain chemistry to mental illness" (p. 3). He continues: "the claim that psychotherapeutic drugs correct a chemical imbalance that is the root cause of most psychological problems also rests on a very shaky scientific foundation" (p. 3). And, again:

> There are good reasons for believing that every psychological state is influenced by different neurotransmitters and by brain circuits distributed widely throughout the brain that undoubtedly involve a number of different neurotransmitters. Furthermore, all information available should lead us to conclude that every neurotransmitter and every receptor target plays a role in different behavioral and psychological phenomena. (p. 5)

We have been faced with numerous examples of this attempt to establish and exploit a very large financial market that reflects the widespread presence of psychological problems and the vulnerability of this particular population to the mirage of a "chemical" cure behind which to hide the reluctance for self-exploration and self-disclosure. Furthermore, a purely "chemical imbalance" exonerates the subjects from any perception of guilt or shame. In a previous footnote I pointed to the present push for antidepressants to become drugs for multiple use. TV advertisements show flashy synaptic clefts and seductive invitations to use a particular agent in order to restore a person's happiness and well-being.[3]

Many in the field recall a famous book on Prozac (Kramer, 1993/1997). The author gave the common reader the impression that the drug could sculpt the

---

[3] Indeed, the list of "symptoms" flashed on our screens by pharmaceutical companies advertising their products is quite encompassing and it disregards important aspects such as severity and symptom clusters, so that everyone sad or temporarily distressed might feel justified in using the chemical rather than addressing his or her relationship to the vicissitudes of life; the advertisements also lack information regarding the array of collateral consequences from the pervasive and cascading effects of the agent.

Multiple sclerosis

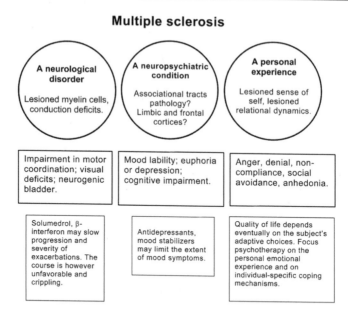

Figure 11-3: The hierarchical spectrum of multiple sclerosis.

personality and went so far as to question whether such "cosmetic psychophar-macology" should be ethically acceptable. Unfortunately the situation is quite far from the one so heavily advertised. The fantasy that the social complexities caused by the Bin Ladens of our times could be magically and permanently erased with some Prozac is sheer nonsense.

Neuroscience will eventually come to represent the most essential aspect of human knowledge; it is imperative that it protects itself from the impingement of other territorial demands, so that it can continue to be our crucial tool toward the understanding of psyche rather than being seduced or bought into becoming a tool of power and economics.

The following vignettes will reinforce the three-dimensional view of psy-chiatric treatment.

AP, a single (divorced) woman in her early forties, had been diagnosed 10 years earlier with multiple sclerosis (MS). CF is a single (divorced) man of a similar age who was also diagnosed 10 years earlier with MS. Both cases present a condition that emerges out of dynamic phenomena at multiple levels of the hierarchy. At the left of Figure 11-3 molecular factors affect neural membranes and eventuate in complex deficits in neurotransmission, scattered in an unstable way at different sites of the central nervous system. The central column represents dynamics occurring within assemblies and systems of assemblies affected by the disturbance in neurotransmission. The right column can be conceptualized as emerging out of mental dynamics that operate at the upper levels of the hierarchy, including cultural factors. In the case of multiple sclerosis, psychopharmacotherapy has no effect on the primary deficit in neurotransmission but may play a significant role in dampening disturbances reflecting the downward effect from the "feeling of what happens" related to the subjective experience of the physical disability. It may also play a substantial role in counteracting to some extent the "mood" side effects from the chemotherapeutic agents and from other pharmacological interventions as intermittent high-dosage steroid administration. One needs, however, to be alert and able to differentiate cognitive and affective changes secondary to reactive psychological states such as depression and anxiety from primary declines in cognitive and affective function caused by specific associational tracts disease.

The cases of AP and GF poignantly illustrate similarities as well as differences. One can reasonably assume that at the level of the primary disorder in the myelin cells the disease of these two brains was very similar, despite the variables in their developmental selection. The assumption can be extended to the next higher levels of the hierarchy, given that the distribution of the lesions does stochastically favor specific systems, and the clusters of symptoms (motoric, ocular, visceral) did not differ in any substantial way. At the upper levels of the hierarchy, however, the disease of the organ becomes also and predominantly the subject's experience of an illness. Out of the dynamics of this experience the experience of living emerges. And here the two cases differed in substantial ways.

At these upper levels, the experience of the illness becomes quite influenced by sociocultural factors that have been articulated as collective value systems, which may eventuate in profoundly different adaptive outcomes. Psychotherapy deals primarily with these complex dynamics and their emergent products that ultimately encapsulate the membrane disorder and its physical correlates. AP, aware of the "miniaturization of my life"—as she aptly put it—caused by the physical limitations, anchored herself to a strong belief in an unaffected cognition and to a perceived demand from her parental, social, and cultural systems that she cope with the disease and the progressive diminution in body and self-identity by remaining loyal to the rule of seeking an "honorable" way. Suicide was utterly unacceptable and sinful. She sought further education and kept busy with plans that were frequently unrealistic (as were the ongoing expectations from her subculture) but gave her a sense of control over her otherwise helpless state.

Gifted with emotional acuity, her affective responses were intense and often quite painful to experience, but she kept a very conservative approach to antidepressants once she had experienced their muting effect and always chose to feel "more rather than less."[4]

CF, on the contrary, was emotionally constricted and could not extricate himself from the loss in territoriality and dominance that accompanied his experience of the illness. This attitude found reinforcement in the familial and cultural background that mandated male accomplishments and despised any manifestations of "weakness" and of "sissy" emotionality. Failure to perform along these mandates was perceived not only as a failure toward the family values but also toward the values of his subculture. Unable to find a logical explanation, and unable to empathically connect for support, he drifted into heavy alcohol abuse that would allow for explosions of rage for which he could avoid taking any ownership ("alcohol talks"). In lieu of creative connections with the feelings emanating from his wounded self he sought solace by immersing himself in the home viewing of endless movies, largely of war and violence, that probably acted as the projections of the unaccepted emotional package triggered by his experiencing the illness. His sporadic and brief encounters with treatment were dense with sarcasm and statements that everything was "fine."

KN offers a closing vignette of the hyperimmense number of variables inherent to the cognitive hierarchy and to the phase space of mind. A middle-aged woman with three adult and very successful children, she suffered from severe obsessive–compulsive disease (OCD), its unrecognized precursors reaching far back into her childhood and early adolescence. Five years of "pure" psychotherapy had brought only a mild and temporary amelioration of her crippling disorder. When seen at this present phase of therapy she scored very high on all OC scales and admitted so much pain that she wished she would die (her religion, which represented for her a fundamental center of being, strongly condemned suicide).

A new psychotherapeutic trial was begun, but this time she was also treated from the very beginning with high doses of the most effective "anti-OCD" medication available, augmented up to her limits of tolerance by adjunctive agents. Over the months the intensity of some symptoms started to recede and in her second year of treatment (characterized also by psychotherapy along two themes: the ongoing confrontation of the illogicality of her "rules" and an exploration of some core inflexible traits of her personality) she could report a 50% improvement.

---

[4] The affective richness fostered an equally rich propensity for analogical thinking. Many of these "unexpected associations" and similes were only superficially anchored to external reality and had to be relinquished; but several others offered creative alternatives and were truly adaptive.

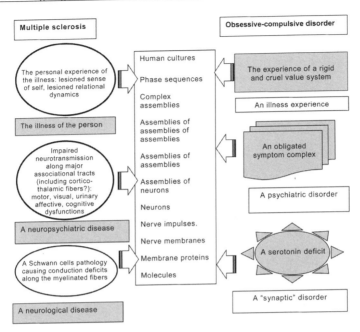

Figure 11-4: The disease—illness spectrum along the hierarchy of cognitive dynamics.

Then a grandchild was born and she came to take care of him 1 day a week. During that day she would regularly be symptom free, in a relaxed and joyful mood, fully and freely invested in the loving relationship with the child (the care of her own children had caused profound distress and frequent attacks of paralyzing anxiety).

Admittedly, despite my acute interest, therapy has not been able to identify and exploit the powerful attractor that, 1 day a week, transforms this subject and heals her psyche. But I cannot refrain from recalling the wounded Psyche of the myth, mourning for her lost (or never tasted) happiness, and the healing power of Eros. Apuleius would probably be puzzled and amused by my inability to understand and accept the depth and the "self-evident" dynamics of KN's *metamorphosis*!

Figure 11-4 summarizes the different emergent outcomes in the disease–illness continuum, and how the perspective and the understanding may change with the observer remaining focused to a specific level of abstraction. When plotted against the hierarchical levels and conceptualized in the trilingual model expounded throughout the book, the conditions assume a different definition and their landscapes become truly multidimensional.

Chapter 12

THE PSYCHOTHERAPEUTIC DIALOGUE: INTERSUB-JECTIVITY

The case of KN is a poignant example of the intricacy of the dynamics that operate within a mental space: loops of recursive causation, often unimaginable, and hidden powerful attractors that become activated into existence out of their potential condition, to provoke compelling emergent outcomes while remaining themselves completely out of, or perhaps just at the fringes of ego consciousness; and then quickly fading again into a "dispositional configuration" (Damasio, 1999) until the next reactivation. In KN's case we encounter rigidly set patterns of "serotonin dysfunction" built upon a primary, "genetic" state of synaptic dysregulation or as epigenetic sets of misfiring neural maps; the compulsion is perceived as a profoundly painful experience that is totally ego alien and hated by the subject because it consumes her psyche and robs her of most of her life. Still, no amount of logical thinking, even if repeated over and over, could have any effect whatsoever on the obligated behavior, nor do the subject's hate and anguish. A flooding with high doses of "serotonin regulators" is partially successful at best. But one day a week something different flourishes in the subject: a motus cordis, a movement of the heart, a feeling of peace and freedom born out of the healing love for a child in a mind which has in the past experienced profound, but unhealing, love for her own children. This factor requires interactional attributes (because it is effective only when the child is physically present) in order to emerge from invisible dynamics at the upper levels of KN's cognitive hierarchy. When activated it erases or "corrects" the synaptic dysregulation and the metastable maps and it represents a very strong, indisputable example of downward causation.

It is entirely possible that such temporary erasure could emerge only because of the reduction in the severity of the neurochemical dysfunction realized by the use of the medications; however, the effectiveness and the flexibility of the response to the unknown correcting factor strongly amend any possible scientific myth of a purely anatomically based "chemical imbalance" to represent the single explanation for the disorder.

It is also telling that, although the composite attractor has been clearly recognized into the ego consciousness of both subject and therapist, and although its emotional package represents a distinct and experientially alive memory that KN can reevoke with ease, the truly effective causal element has escaped conscious recognition. The therapy has not been able to identify it and transform it into an enduring healing experience that would continue even when the child is not "there." Do other sensory modalities require participation? Which library does KN visit? Which book is taken off the shelf? This is a fitting example of the formidable task of psychotherapy in its search for that unique copy of common themes, for the hidden key to open a detour to other landscapes. Indeed, someone said that psychotherapists are skilled in creating detours in the brain.

The diversion requires, however, that the mental universe of the subject be respected. Therapy has great powers, among which the power to create virtual realities that reflect the therapist's mind and in the short run could be quite effective (comparable to the experience of falling in love with a set of e-mails) but eventually would backfire. When dealing with the mind of another person proper therapy is required to intersubjectively connect with a domain comparable in complexity to our own and to assist in extracting and clarifying the contextual issues as they are expressed by means of analogies that represent the first-person language of that specific mind. In my opinion the process requires that the therapist assumes a different standing in his or her relationship with the subject than the one emerging from the traditional conceptualization of the self-other relationship. A few statements on intersubjectivity are therefore in order and I will briefly use a few of the poignant arguments from the writings of Jessica Benjamin (1998).

The term *intersubjectivity* was introduced by Stolorow (1987) to mean a field of intersection of two subjectivities. Benjamin expands on Stolorow's definition and points to the difference between perceiving the other as objec-tified—an object separate from us, that has actually been expelled from our intrapsychic world—and the other perceived as a subject, a center of being equivalent to us and interconnected to us in complex ways. Benjamin points out (and I hope I am not oversimplifying her line of reasoning) that the exclusive focus on the need to differentiate from the original "mother-object"—and to cast such internal representation outside the self and into the position of a true "object" from which we are required to separate and to individuate—actually misses the fact that prior to the disavowal the primary "object" was a part of the inner world and a partner to it "It was, in short, *a concrete other in a reciprocal relationship where each constitutes the other*" (Benjamin, 1998, p. 89): a true closed causal loop!

She postulates a developmental process of connectedness in the intersubjective dimension that counterpoints the development of separation-identification
in the intrapsychic dimension. The first process entails a capacity for *mutual
recognition* that is only gradually and imperfectly acquired: a need to be
recognized as well as the capacity to recognize the other. She suggests that
the intersubjective dimension of the analytic encounter should be reframed
as "where objects were, subjects must be." In her opinion, the difference
between the other as an object and the other as a subject is crucial to relational
psychotherapy. The subtle shift within the analyst in experiencing the other as
an equal subject (although not identical to the self!) is in my opinion crucial
to erasing the equally subtle tension that becomes energized in the effort of
maintaining the self as separate from the other/nonself. Out of this tension a
tendency may emerge, "to force the other to either be or want what it (the
subject) wants, to assimilate the other.... It is the extension of reducing the
difference to sameness, the inability to recognize the other without dissolving
her/his otherness" (Benjamin, 1998, p. 86).

Only when operating from this position can the therapist visit the landscape
of the subject and relate to its vistas in an intersubjective way, without the
risk of inferring or suggesting conclusions extracted from his or her own
landscapes. It took Apuleius over 100 pages to describe the dynamic-genetic
formulation of his Psyche and her therapeutic journey toward integration. It was
a journey that included a phase of unsuccessful search for resolution outside of
the self until eventually she underwent the traditional and predictable descent
into the personal hell of the symptoms complex and of the ghosts and fearful
images and memories that populate the unconscious. It is a process that unfolds
within the confines of the subject's uniqueness; it is frequently accompanied
by fears that by going there one may "lose my mind," lose the grasp on
conscious rationality and succumb to some "disordered state," become lost,
mad. Requests for reassurance and inquiries about the therapist's "knowing"
and having a script of the entire process are very routine at this stage of
treatment. The same fear may echo within the psyche of the therapist and it
may trigger attempts to actively contain it by designing what in the therapist's
mind is a "safe" set of dynamics, an intellectual and logical sequence of events.
The real task and skill required at this point are to reduce the anguish stemming
from separateness through intersubjective support, while avoiding carrying the
support to an excess. Excessive support may foster a partial identification with
the therapist and transform the subject into a "therapist I" or a component of
that I, by incorporating the therapist's expectation and vision.

A truly integrated psychotherapy requires some awareness and understanding of the hierarchical systems from which the subject's experiences emerge;
we can then find guidance in empathy and intuition as tools that can help us to
follow the broad relationships of causality operative among the different levels.

Another crucial element in performing intersubjective psychotherapy has to deal first with the recognition of the libraries of knowledge in ourselves; only then may we recognize some common themes in the subject, albeit disguised by his or her idiosyncratic adaptation. One needs to remember the existence of the database and be conciliatory toward the immensity of the themes; Pratchett's reminder of the ape on top of the rat that stands on the lizard may sound irreverent and fictional but is actually quite realistic. Much "strange" human behavior becomes clearer—or at least open to a different understanding—once the evolutionary hierarchy is included as a consideration of causality. Consider the interconnection between the evolutionary themes of dominance and sexuality in the phenotype of male primacy. In the mammal kingdom male alpha dominance extends to include the territory and the opposite gender. Within a specific group, subordination is often signaled through a ritualistic sexual subjugation—the dominant figure acting out a "mating" behavior and the weaker "other" signaling acceptance by a submissive sexual behavior. Wherever sexuality is expressively linked to competition and dominance, it will then be played out along these lines; therefore, it is not uncommon for a mammal male, as a lion, not belonging to the pride and seeking acceptance and admission to it, to attempt sexual possession upon an established female of the "tribe" as a signature of his request. When seen against this piece of evolutionary information the act of rape may carry a more complex and tragic meaning (as an archaic response to a state of exclusion and "not belonging" rather than a shallow "sexual predator" description, which still does not clarify the causative loops) with roots emerging already at the origin of the species, from prehuman evolutionary dynamics.[1] Our journey into the landscape of a rapist should require the visiting of these evolutionary scenarios and how they became entangled in the subject's epigenetic and developmental vicissitudes. The recognition of such a scenario as a common inheritance that we too share may facilitate a therapeutic encounter that otherwise could be emotionally complex and possibly adversarial.[2]

Another dilemma arising from the psychotherapeutic interactions carried out in the intersubjective domain may be contained in Cornell's (1992) statement: "The strangeness of the Other is that the Other is an 'I'. But, as an 'I', the Other is the same as 'me'" (p. 57). The simultaneous coexistence of the connectedness theme counterbalances and accompanies individuation. This intricate set of value systems constitutes the "attractor" represented by the inner companion (or parent, or [M]other, or adversary) illustrated in Figure 12-1.

---

[1] Recall Figure 7-2, p. 76.

[2] A component of the adversarial response in a male therapist could even express his countertransference stemming from his unconscious recognition of the challenge to his own dominance implied in the rape of a female belonging to his social "pride."

We may call it a complex, a conflict, a state of mind, "the discourse of the Other" in Lacanian terms, the shadow of the other (Benjamin), the stranger in us (Kristeva) or any other way we choose.

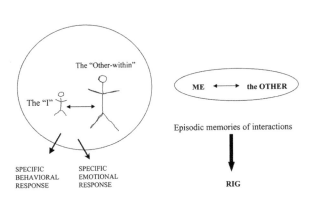

SPECIFIC BEHAVIORAL RESPONSE   SPECIFIC EMOTIONAL RESPONSE   RIG

Figure 12-1: The "other" within.

The diagram expressed on the left side of Figure 12-1 finds its expression through specific behavioral manifestations and emotional states, and it represents an inevitable composite internal configuration that finds its origin in the state of affairs of an object that is also, originally, the subject. I am of the opinion that the original imprinting of the first "other" in the self is a normal, necessary, inevitable evolutionary process, essential to survival. Its roots are very ancient, running through the programs of parental bonding as it appeared at a certain point in evolution. The imprinting of a newborn zebra to the unique stripe pattern of the mother takes place immediately after birth; within an hour the newborn will be able to identify and follow its mother's stripes throughout a night stampede from attacking carnivores, when the entire scenario is just a universe of running stripes, flashing away in the darkness. It is just one example—more stunning than others perhaps—of a pattern of relationship between the self and the "big other" that is shared by multiple species and includes the experience of each one of us. There is a very crucial, actually vital aspect in the other and in its relationship to the newborn, emerging biological being; and there is an evolutionary demand that it be internalized. In the zebra this internalization seems to consist in a concrete affective visualization; in minds at a more complex evolutionary level the internalization will acquire increased abstraction and symbolic status (a process similar to the evolution of the territoriality theme discussed earlier on). We carry this "other-within-us" as an imprinted image of the primary source of life and safety and order: not purely as an individualized psychological event but *as an evolutionary biological necessity*: a true archetypal construct in a Jungian sense. The template imposes that its dictates, its unique stripes, are to be followed; they are life-saving; if we get disconnected we get lost and will not survive.

Such primal connectedness[3] tends to lose its compelling quality as the individual self matures and seeks autonomy, and other learning, such as mastery and self-reliance, takes place and fosters individualized versions of the value systems of the other within. When a dissonance persists and complicates the ownership of values—their adaptation to the subject's overall position concerning life—then the therapist is faced with a clinical syndrome. In the diagram on the right side of Figure 12-1, excessive persistence and control from the actual other transform episodic memories of a specific type of connectedness into representations of interactions that become generalized (RIG); these patterns can be conceptualized as Hebbian learning effect, as metastable assemblies, or splintered dynamic cores, or attractors, or unconscious dynamics. They maintain at least some of the compelling quality of the imprinting phenomenon, color the sense-of-the-self-in-the-world, and become played out in the intersubjective domain of significant relationships, including therapy and its intersubjective process.[4] The therapist's recognition of the subject-object tension, and the ability for self-empathy (experienced in the countertransference and in the projective identifications that might mirror in the external world what is an internal event) can then be translated into how a person perceives her or his role within the composite landscape.

CH, a 30-year-old widow, came to her first session one year after the death of her husband from brain cancer. She had recent-onset panic attacks. She reported that after his death she went to see one therapist but he felt very moved by her history and "I couldn't stand his feelings and did not want sympathy;" so she did not go back. This created an interesting dilemma: if I "felt," she would withdraw, if I did not feel, I would withdraw; both options appeared to be countertherapeutic: the "she-the-other" suggested that I remain unemotional as she appeared to prefer; it was after all her husband, not mine; the "she-the-subject," however, required my recognition in myself and in her of her experience. I sensed the strong tension between connectedness and separation, which could suggest a conflict with the other within; but nothing else was visible, in the intersubjective landscape. Perhaps she did not want to be involved again with another person's suffering.

It seemed crucial that she perceive mutual *recognition* of her emotional experience. It seemed equally important that she be shielded from the risk of *emotional identification*: her feelings, and suffering, becoming my feelings, and suffering. I commented that I could not be expected to erase my deep empathy

---

[3] The evolutionary role and the developmental nature of connectedness clarify its appropriateness in therapy.

[4] This two-character setting, in which the ego represents the lesser one, is a very frequent clinical finding loaded with potent affects; once identified, the names given by the subject to the other-within can be quite telling: the "Taskmaster," the "Censor," the "Executioner."

for the frightening experience of her husband's slow death, but evidently I would not feel what she did; perhaps she could recognize my empathy while not responding to a requirement that she protects me from hurting, that she take care of me too. She verbalized "relief," dwelt on the last few months of her husband's illness, the horror of seizures, mental obtundation, incontinence, and loss of any ability for self-care, end-of-treatment options, and finally his death in her lap. She felt guilty that maybe she had not done all that she could have done for him. She scheduled another appointment, *one month* later.

She spent this appointment discussing how deeply she had emotionally resonated with the movie *A Beautiful Mind*. The wife's role brought her repeatedly to tears. She had also felt cheated, she did not understand why. It had been a profound and moving experience.

I was impressed and perplexed by her ego's apparent inability to see the glaring similarity between the two wives and the diversity in outcomes, so I abstained from comments. She described the session as helpful and scheduled a third appointment. This time she spoke about a new boyfriend. He was nice, but she was afraid he may not be dependable as he kept quitting jobs. He was also controlling and put a lot of demands upon her. She asked me: "Should I dump him and be a quitter and feel guilty for that?" Again, I was faced with a request without "good" outcomes: I was asked either to promote distancing and guilt or closeness and dependence. But this time I thought I saw an emerging pattern. I shared how I felt dysfunctional (my problem) and unable to satisfy her request; I wondered if she felt destined to depend on, and perhaps take care of, dysfunctional people: her husband, the beautiful mind, her boyfriend, and me.

Her response was an affect link: she cried and talked about her lifelong relationship with a dysfunctional and controlling, never satisfied mother whom she loved deeply. She recognized the configuration of Figure 12-1 as going on in her mind all the time. She started to schedule weekly sessions.

To be most effective, the translation that the therapist proposes should be presented in the language of the subject, because this is the language that facilitates internal connectedness with the personal history and the affective domain. The therapist's ability to empathically connect to the language of the subject and recognize its metaphors and complex meanings facilitates a keener understanding of the other. Even more crucial, our ability to use it generates in the other the feeling of being understood (the mutual recognition process postulated by Benjamin). Its use therefore permits a dialogue in which an entire scenario could be brought into the picture without having to use an artificial list of all its components. The feelings attached to the metaphors permeate the interaction and become alive; both "subjects" truly operate within the same mental space, within the same "feeling of what happens."

I had mentioned (p. 88) how PD used the terms *going south* (and *going north*) to convey a very complex scenario. It included affective and behavioral configurations, the contraposition between his biological father, who had died when he was a child, and his stepfather; his relationship to sexuality and to his needs from others; and intricate, often antithetic systems of values. These were his metaphors that the therapist was eventually able to recognize within his own mind as "subject-to-subject." In the therapist the metaphors emerged out of different conglomerates of variables but also carried some common meaning that could be shared in the intersubjective dimension to validate the subject's experience, generate in him the sense of having been correctly recognized, and allow for some reframing of its causative elements.

The witnessing of these experiences and the language of the subject inevitably transforms the therapist. While this transformation need not be permanent—its persistence beyond the encounter frequently manifests itself in some sort of role confusion or boundary violation—it can be very significant in allowing a real participation to the scene or pattern that is played out.

Chapter 13

THE ROLE OF A NEW SCIENCE FOR PSYCHE UPON SOCIETY AND CULTURE

I addressed in Chapter 10 the need for a new scientific paradigm to understand biological life, including mind. Such a shift is essential because the mind is where our culture and society reside, and it is my strong opinion that our insistence on remaining ignorant about the mind of humanity, out of looking at it from the wrong perspective, is highly responsible for the way in which we perpetuate the tragic aspects of our mode of being alive as a species, as social groups, and as individuals.

The comments that follow do not address global issues about which I have only a limited understanding; others have studied and written on the theme of civilization and its discontent to great depths and with impressive and still inspiring insights. I want simply to offer a few comments on the relationship that a science of mind, and the understanding of the three languages, has with the culture and the social order, and with the structuring of Dawkins' memes. The relationship appears to me to be at present often lopsided, or stultified by a lack of correspondence between its elements.

I indicated how, when faced with a process of research and with a language that is not imbued with the "neutral" and "essential" mode of expression of scientific materialism, many researchers snub it as "frivolous" and inconsequential.[1] Yet, most of the mental activity and language attributable to humanity has the characteristics of being not at all neutral but rather deeply centered on choices and values, and of promoting difference and irregularity rather than duplication and reliability. The artificial language of "research" on the human mind is not really human, and most of its users and supporters would never use it outside of their laboratories and institutes of research. This phenomenon is quite puzzling; it is as if the study of a specific biological organism in its

---

[1] I have, though, already quoted earlier [p. 8] Wallace's observation concerning the inevitable link of "objective" science to the motus cordis of its society and culture.

natural habitat would be considered not illustrative and misleading, so that its study under those conditions should give precedence to an exclusive laboratory situation.

Science therefore is at a loss in explaining multiple aspects of the culture and its social order. Consider for a moment the following short report.[2] "Vatican: a step toward sainthood." The Vatican office ... authenticated a miracle attributed to Mother Theresa of Calcutta. ... The miracle was the healing of a stomach tumor in an Indian woman who had prayed to the nun" (Bruni, 2002, p. A4).

Scientific materialism sits very uncomfortably with this type of teasers. They create unwanted turbulence and disturb the proper order of events. The progressive mechanical view of the universe that had begun to emerge in the 16th century put a lid on anything that sounded "magical" and it joined forces with the Protestant reformers. "By the nineteenth century, religion in the West had come to be strongly associated with Romanticism: it dealt with matters of the heart, leaving matters of the intellect to science and philosophy.... And science ... gradually came to ignore religion on the grounds that it is intrinsically private, subjective, and even irrational in nature" (Wallace, 2000, p. 55). Therefore Christian theology became compelled to differentiate true miracles, due to God, from plain marvels of nature, and it turned to science in order to define the laws of nature and allow for the identification of true miracles because these could not be explained by the natural laws of scientific materialism. When the Church of Rome states that Mother Theresa performed a miracle it explicitly states that what happened falls outside the laws of science; implicitly it proclaims other sets of divine laws and, in the case of a physical event such as a tumor, it implies a sort of dualism that understandably does not have a chance of being accepted in a materialistic vision of the world.

The non-Catholic scientist may frown or suppress an inner condescending smile or just plainly think no more of it. The Catholic scientist may undergo a subliminal split between the scientist and the devout believer, or may silently "dismiss" the event to the realm of "Divine Providence": to an intervention of the God. (These interventions have been much more rare than before, since humanity codified what miracles were and are.) The general Western scientist may also reflect that:[3]

---

[2] I am very grateful to synchronicity and to Mother Theresa for providing me with this vignette, which stands smack in the center of the main Western religious cultural value system, and carries the imprimatur of the number 1 Ecclesia, a structure utterly incapable of lies. If I had to resort to some example out of the Eastern cultures—as I thought I would be obliged to—my point would have been more dismissible as "another eastern fancy."

[3] Evidently I am not *actually speaking* for all Western scientists. If the reader does not find his or her response among the ones listed below it simply means that my empathic processes are limited, as indeed they are.

- "Spontaneous" healing of malignancies is a natural event and not an indication of Divine intervention.
- Tumor is too generic a term; it includes benign forms and other spontaneously reversible conditions. And, can we trust the Indian diagnostic skills? After all aren't they rather "behind us," technologically (we shall be magnanimous and not whisper, even to our selves, any skepticism about their scientific standing)?
- The Catholic Church—at the local, Indian level as well as in Rome—has to have a vested interest, as well as a fascination with promoting saints (its major representatives) and through them its own goodness, particularly during these troubled times when it totters under so many strains and scandals.

Unspoken and not addressed are some interesting points:

1. The recognized status of the Catholic Church protects it from being called psychotic or a malingerer. Scientific dissent is expressed respectfully and with great consideration being given to the fact that the Church represents a Divinity (even if I do not believe in it) and a good part of humanity. Yet, the concept and the documentable scientific substance of a "miracle" are not different from my telling that I spoke with aliens through the intergalactic void. What explains this implicit acceptance? What psychological functions support such a profound, pervasive set of values and meanings that continue to replicate ancient symbols such as the Sahu and the Sekhem, as well as their interactive state in the subject's Osiris? What does science omit to study when it disconnects itself from any analysis of these generalized attributes of being human?

2. "Spontaneous" resolution of tumors has indeed happened. What does science brush away when it uses the term spontaneous? What is the true psychobiology supporting these rather rare and unnatural events?

In my opinion an uneasy alliance has stemmed out of the interplay between these two aspects of culture, religion and science, that prefer to maintain a conventional status[4] rather than to truly enlighten humanity by seeking the meaning behind the phenomenon. The outcome is that the educational process of the culture is deprived of its psychological dimension: the complexity of the human mind is not considered a pertinent topic for education because either it could disturb the dogmas upon which religion rests, or it could disturb the dogmas upon which science rests. Furthermore, both religion and science are strongly courted by politics that assume through them legitimacy and support, and pay them back in the same coin.

---

4 "Traditional forms of religion have been reduced to socially acceptable formulas with which to embellish a life that has been made comfortable by science and technology" (Wallace, 2000, p. 55).

The outcome is a society and a culture that are psychologically illiterate. Humans do not have any real sense of the profundity and intricacy of their minds, nor are they taught to identify the streams of collective data and affective states that participate in their own being. The importance for a redefinition of consciousness as outlined in Chapter 5 is based on the fact that it reinstates the substantial role that non-ego consciousness plays in the process of living; it is therefore essential that we study it in detail, along with ways to improve global knowledge (at a social and cultural level) and to improve the communication between ego and self, and our knowledge of how this communication works.

The importance of this process, which reinstates at a social level the Socratic "know thyself," is quite evident all around us: when individuals lack sufficient autonomy and ego-self integration, the logic of the collective bends to the emotional tone and to the system of values that it is being fed with. Suicide bombers and terrorism are powerful examples of a "rational," "logical" way of processing reality that is actually driven by raw affects. The ego of the social system is not equipped to master emotional surges by a correct understanding of its primal, instinctual origins (like the perception of profound threats to one's survival), but it is rather captured by them, and its logical power is bent to the service of the heightened affect. This state of affairs replicates in the social dimension the individual scenario seen in psychotherapy and characterized by disconnectedness between self and ego.

Concomitantly to the dark side of psychological illiteracy contained in "the adversary image" we witness an equally dangerous white side in the phenomenon of the hero-leaders who promulgate the "rightful" exercise of dominance, without having any recognition of their inner landscape and of the instinctual nature of their ego-conscious actions. Dominance and territoriality continue to be the driving variables, intertwined with more personal themes such as competition with the "other within," intersubjective immaturity (inability to perceive the other outside as a subject too, similar to the "I," rather than as an alien to be split off from the "I"), and disconnectedness from the low-focus realm of spirituality (Gelertner, 1994, pp. 91–98).

In Chapter 9 I hinted at a developmental path in which humanity could play a causal part rather than allowing for chance events to mold future psychological changes. Several steps were suggested, beginning with the need for an expanded acceptance and recognition of the richness and role of unconscious dynamics (as well as their archaic origins) upon the ego's conscious state. This sort of information has to be distributed in an organized and robust way so that it can achieve a social acceptance. The "dark" sides of the biological organism need to be understood as complementing necessities that have or had their adaptive value. The archaic, prehuman nature of many aspects of the database has to be illuminated.[5] The experience from psychotherapy illustrates the readiness of individuals to learn about the intricacy of their minds, and to discover a personal domain until then unexpected and surprising, as the staterooms of the palace were to Psyche. It also demonstrates how an expanded knowledge of the mind can direct the reframing of values and the modulation of emotions. Only when this phase of acknowledgment is achieved could one begin to focus on how to optimize the channels of communication between the self and the ego, so that the unconscious richness of evolutionary experience can be reliably and knowingly tapped into, and used to negotiate our interactive reality.

Another decisive step in this developmental outline is the sociocultural focus on the gradual development of truly mature values that would foster an intersubjective perception of the other. These systems could gradually mitigate the patterns of territoriality and dominance, and become a crucial part of the knowledge upon which the brain acts: a verily major educational task of integrated efforts at all levels of social interactions: family, school, media, law, politics, economy, human rights and so on.

The task of mastering the power of the primal affects present within each mind, and to educate humanity in order to enhance the evolutionary chances by influencing the knowledge upon which the future brain will act, will be very hard—the myth of Psyche illustrates quite well how hard it may be. In the following pages I will examine few specific themes contained within the immense libraries of knowledge upon which the brain operates: the aggressive drive and its related templates of phenotypic male primacy, dominance, and territoriality. Throughout the years I have given particular clinical and cross-cultural attention to these themes and to how they affect the cognitive dynamics of individuals and of groups—and, by extrapolation, of social systems and cultures. These themes are linked to the other psychological developmental processes that also frame the human interactive dynamics: either autonomy

---

[5] Again, it is easy to find examples of the archaic roots for the stunning removal of connectedness when the other becomes a competing entity and is ejected from "our" rightful territory (and in this way the nice "neighbor" becomes the communist, the radical, the liberal, the atheist, the terrorist, Asian, African, Muslim). One may simply follow Darwin to the Galapagos and observe how, when food is scarce, the Sulae Nebouxi (Blue-footed boobies) offspring will compete for food and for territory. Once a weaker chick is pushed outside of the white guano circle that represents a symbol of the nest, (the equivalent of a line in the sand) the parents themselves *will not recognize it anymore* as their offspring, and will stop feeding it. The lines from Pratchett that I reported earlier on about an intellect a billion years old were inserted deliberately, as a piece of scientific observation; in its archipallium, paleopallium, and neopallium subdivisions the brain carries the lizard and the mouse, and the ape. Science needs to start and "imagine what comes out of the dark places, (when) uncontrolled(?)" The knowledge of the dark places needs to be recognized and controlled, harnessed toward psychological growth.

obtained through expulsion of the other from our psychic territory, or enduring connectedness with recognition of the other as a subject similar to us.

History shows that human cultures have proven a great ability for unsurpassed aggressivity and a rapacious appetite for ever-expanding territories of all kinds. A profound reevaluation of the male phenotype is required, and constraints have to be developed upon its driving aspects: dominance, territoriality, and sexuality seem to act as a package in the expression of male aggressivity. The systematized rapes of the females of the other during the Bosnian wars is just one of innumerable examples on this theme. It is located at an extreme of a spectrum that includes, near the opposite pole, more standard expressions of the same trend, as the benevolent neglect toward sexual abuse of women characteristic of the patriarchal military systems, as well as the forceful preoccupation of males for maintaining decisional power upon the women's reproductive system.[6] A reformulation of aggressivity, an indisputable biological drive with its own survival function, and its elaboration into more mature expressions as assertiveness, could significantly defuse and contain the present prevalence of archaic, unadulterated violence; this process could be substantially enhanced by a greater understanding of the connectedness drive and by an increased recognition of the other as a subject, as an "as I."

Overall humanity is probably not more violent and pathologically aggressive toward other groups than it has been since the Homeric age of the great palaces. My point is that our acknowledgment that humans are by far the most destructive species on the planet does not justify our continuing to be so. Humanity is, "arguably without doubt" gifted with an expanding mental apparatus that is probably unequalled in the entire planet. It can blindly accept an evolutionary progression of Psyche based on chance phenomena or it can decide to use its ability for knowledge in the service of molding future knowledge and, through this last process, evolution itself. As Nobelian Jimmy Carter said, violence might be necessary at times, but it is always evil, and psychologically regressive; the idea of fostering peace by war has been the routinely attempted solution to territorial and dominance problems since men found themselves in a state of conflict with other men. It never worked; at best it repressed the conflict for a while, as in Communist Russia. Even the Pax Romana was kept by the endless use of massive patrolling armies and it ended with the fragmentation of Roman military power.

The three "pillars of civilization," science, religion, and the politics of the capitalistic state, have often been at odds with each other but have shown a

---

[6] Religion is not exempt from rewarding male aggression with sex, from the Valkyrs tending the slain heroes in the warrior hall of the god Odin to the Muslim Huri, the blue-eyed givers of tender care to the true God-warrior; neither is myth, as the oedipal family tragedy indicates.

tendency to collude into negating those aspects of the subject that do not fit their vision of the world. The terms themselves have acquired a life and a psychic consistency of their own, as if they were indeed true realities rather than the articulation of human endeavors. In this sense the modern human has been subjected to molding by these systems of power, thus reflecting the antisubjective opinions of Foucault and Butler that we briefly visited in Chapter 2. All these three systems have been very invested in the status of their dominance and have often recurred to their subject(s)' constitutional potential for aggressivity in order to enforce such dominance. The philosophy that the protection of the God/state-parent justifies aggression becomes a dogma that is instilled in the subject with the first breath; to differ from it puts the subject in opposition with powerful sets of values, a strong psychological "attractor" that will put constraints on creative thought production, will generate in the ego images of deviating from the system, and will threaten the subject's need for connectedness and recognition.

Even the leaders of today's three pillars of civilization are often possessed by the drives in a primal way, and overtly insensitive to, and incapable of, psychological depth and enlightened self-empathy. They exist and operate merely within the narrow confines of ego consciousness and would not know how to identify, analyze, and master the affective drives that mold its rationality. The unmodulated state between ego consciousness and unconscious processes allows for a rationality that is dominated by the drives without the subject being aware of this tragedy but simply "believing" that what "reason" tells is "the right thing."

Furthermore, the power of the capitalist "territory" and economic dominance is very significant; it bends the laws of science—as I have briefly discussed when I reported the influence of economics upon pharmacological research,[7] it pervades the fabric of the churches, and it bends the laws of the legal system too: consider the corporate structure, the disparity in punishment

---

[7] "Dr. David Fleming, ... the disease control centers deputy director for science, (said): 'We try very hard to state objectively what is known ... without nuancing language beyond what is supported by the science' 'Information that used to be based on science,' the lawmakers said, 'is being systematically removed from the public when it conflicts with the administration's political agenda' "(Quoted by Clymer, 2002, p. A17). This systemic altering of scientific information by the political system is even more dramatically outlined in the 2004 report from the Union of Concerned Scientists (www.ucsusa.org), *Restoring Scientific Integrity in Policymaking*, in which over 60 leading scientists—Nobel laureates, leading medical experts, former federal agency directors, and university chairs and presidents—voiced their concern over the misuse of science by the Bush administration.

between "poor" and "rich" crime, the relationship of the political machinery to the law-making process, just to mention a few examples.[8]

A system of ethics has to be developed that would facilitate a gradual diminution of the territoriality and of the dominance themes. As mentioned already, psychotherapy has repeatedly demonstrated how this type of shift in the perception of the human carries profound and enduring maturational gains at the individual level and for all the small social systems, such as families, that have been enriched by an understanding of this dimension, and improve the ability to negotiate with the tension of opposites and with the similarity between the discordant. The documentation from the clinical domain is extremely robust; however, its standing is challenged by the absence of a theoretical scientific framework that would emerge not only from the demotic language of the subjective, but would also find confirmation and modification from the composite alphabet of an integrated neuroscience.

Indeed, science, led by neuroscience, may be called to pick up the guidance in this educational process. Religion may have attempted in the past to foster control over the power of the affective drives by splitting their "dark" side off from the subject and projecting it upon a magical "evil" domain. The repressed material resurfaced in the form of a creed of ownership on the only true divine territory and on the only true God. Therefore, today religion is not the proper educational tool because of its emphasis, at least in the West, on these territorial derivatives (an elected God, an elected doctrine) that put constraints on intersubjectivity with members of different creeds. The Greeks briefly glimpsed at such intersubjective recognition of a common theme in the other, but their philosophy on the matter was lost in the wave of the Judeo-Christian-Islamic apparatus. The political power is equally bound to ignorance of its human psychological assets by the mental distortion that is required for a (democratic) potential leader to become an actual leader: the high focus on power, and on related (Machiavellian) compromises, blunts the ability for analogical thinking and true creativity.

Therefore it seems as if science has to redress its priorities; it must stipulate respectful ethics that favor a different psychological resolution of conflict and postulate the other as another subject; it must find a way to become impervious to the seduction or menace of the present power-oriented systems of social philosophy; it must elaborate a comprehensive design of the psychological and physical mind and of its dynamics along the biological and the cognitive hierarchies; it must convince the social structures of the importance of a psychological education; and it must help these structures in the implementation of the educational program. At a time when science is fascinated with duplication

---

[8] One could adapt to the system of "objective law-making" Wallace's analysis, reported earlier, of the inevitable link between "objective" science and the motus cordis of its society and culture.

of the existing—including human cloning[9]—it could instead focus on the recognition of the difference imbedded in the organization of Psyche, and envision how the knowledge of future brains ought to change and humanity be enriched by the process. Only a new science able to look with great respect at the "poetry" within the human mind could eventually contrive a way to dispel the recurrent disaster of the oedipal crossroads.

The puzzle that opened this book is indeed a magnificent work of knowledge constructed by a structure that is a true tribute to the miracle of life. It contains aspects of my mind that I knew, aspects that I had forgotten, and aspects that I had never realized before. Its content is organized into a powerful and, to me, astounding landscape of my inner self and of its roots into the personal, cultural, and biological libraries. Once faced with the script I was compelled to gradually analyze its meaning and the immensity of the image is stunning. Naturally, one could dismiss it by considering such mental activity stupid or fanatic or romantic or "made up." But, unless that person took a journey inside my mind he or she would never actually know; he or she would simply respond through a logic driven by an emotional package of their own.

A judgment upon the other that is not supported by an intersubjective process fundamentally comes down to represent a mere projection.

Several days after I wrote these last lines,[10] while I was in that state of early morning light sleep in which ego consciousness operates at a very low focus and still floats around in a landscape covered by the mist of sleep, an impressive train of images flashed through the mist. I was driving rather quickly along the ridge of those Boetian hills. Actually, I was not sure if my Alfa was touching the dusty trail or flying low above it. I reached the crossroad. Laius' chariot stood tilted against the hillside, one wheel broken off, two horses still fettered to its pole. Laius laid crumpled on the ground, blood seeping into the dust. Oedipus stood looking down at him, a broad, bloodied sword in his right hand.

"He is your father, Laius," I told him.

"He had to be," he replied, "One cannot escape his own fate that easily."

(Laius made a gurgling sound.)

"Can that chariot of yours fly through time?" he asked.

"I wouldn't know," I answered, "I have never tried."

---

[9] I am not an expert in the intricacies of cloning but the recent flurry of news about the unpredictable and worrisome outcomes made me wonder whether clonation scientists shouldn't give more attention to the caveats found in the hieratic alphabet that I reported previously (Anderson, 1972): the fact that one can now apparently deconstruct the biological organism to a string of codons does not imply that we can use the same string to reconstruct life.

[10] I had spent much time reflecting on the dream and its package was still quite *present* and alive in my mind; as I gradually approached awakening my mind subliminally began to play, on and off, with the images of the puzzle.

We picked up Laius and put him in the back seat of my Alfa. We had to *fold* him a bit, the space there being rather virtual. He looked a little better by the time the folding was completed.

The Alfa landed among tall marble columns on the marbled peristilium of a large Greek temple that was also the entrance of a supermodern hospital. Glass doors slid silently open and young blond barefooted women dressed in white tunics rushed toward us pushing a stretcher.

"Is this Thebes?" I asked Oedipus, as the women transferred Laius to the stretcher.

"In a way it is, and then it is not," he answered: "This is Mount Olympus."

I woke up. I sensed immediately that this set of images offered a closing confirmation of the emergent working of the mind. It was a blueprint of sort, a compressed formula, and actually much of the book could be seen as a downloading in the Ego of the decompressed content of such package.

The dream reverie repeats the message, suggested in the first dream, that the oedipal tragedy may not be inexorable and eternal. The wound is not, as yet, a death wound, although quite severe and "death-like." The potential for other outcomes is still present. It requires the folding of the meaning condensed in the wound—a telling illustration of territoriality and dominance—into a supportive feeling function—the creative connectedness of the (feminine) guiding container—whose true potential has yet to be explored. It also requires that the process can develop the ability to operate along the arch of time and bridge the knowledge disseminated through it. And it requires a scenario in which the Machine is incorporated into the Myth, so to speak, both being consciously acknowledged as expressions of the human spirit.

I would invite the reader to compare these two descriptions of the same mental phenomenon—a quest for modification of the oedipal wound—and reflect on his or her inner response. The first description—the dream—presents the solution in the language of the Self; it emerges out of Self consciousness. The subsequent explanation describes the quest as an intersubjective translation into Ego consciousness of the message from the Self. The first solution is the product of low-focus thinking, suffused with affectivity and rich in images, as well as metaphors and similes; its organization is uniquely subjective (and I tried to reproduce it as precisely as possible), very condensed, and intrinsically obscure to an observer. As one can detect here, the symbolic organization of the Self appears to be based on the construction of an image, which consists in a package of compressed information. Images are usually not communicable—except when captured by the creative insight of true art.

The second solution is presented in the predominantly high-focus, logical language of the Ego. Its affective component has largely evaporated but the message—the image—is now decompressed into words-symbols and becomes open to intersubjective understanding; now it could even satisfy the criteria of scientific psychology. This is the operational mind. At one obscure and largely invisible level of consciousness an incredibly complex structure monitors and directs our survival along neural and mental dynamics fueled by affects, creativity, and what we call spirit. At the other, more transparent and visible level, the same structure further translates the material in a form accessible to Ego exchange. Routinely, we observe and exchange outcomes; we are very rarely witnesses to the underlying process, or fully cognizant of the profound intricacy of its causality. Aside from the neuromental gap, this process of compression and decompression is a truly fascinating one, worth serious investigation.

There is more to the dream, like personal and intimate insights and formulations concerning my individual journey through life. But these aspects may best remain at the periphery of Ego consciousness; indeed, it could be a subtle error to shed too much light on the reframing work to which my Ego had been, briefly, a witness. I feel content and quite safe in just letting myself flow with the stream of my self consciousness, supported by the immensely intricate web of knowledge that resides within my brain.

References

Althusser, L. (1971). *Lenin and Philosophy*. (B. Brewster, Trans.). London: NLB.

American Psychiatric Association. (1994). *Diagnostic and Statistical Manual of Mental Disorders*. Washington, DC.

Anderson, P. W. (1972). More is different: Broken symmetry and the nature of the hierarchical structure of science. *Science, 177*, 393–396.

Apuleius Madaurensis. (1989). *Metamorphoseon*. Cambridge, MA: Harvard University Press.

Arieti, S. (1967). *The Intrapsychic Self: Feeling, Cognition, and Creativity in Health and Mental Illness*. New York: Basic Books.

Aristotle. (1986). *On the Soul*. Cambridge, MA: Harvard University Press.

Asimov, I. (1991). *Second Foundation*. New York: Bantam. (Original work published 1953.)

Benjamin, J. (1998). *Shadow of the Other: Intersubjectivity and Gender in Psychoanalysis*. New York: Routledge.

Bruni, F. (2002, October 2). Vatican: A step toward sainthood. *New York Times*, p. A4.

Budge, E. A. W. (1960). *The Book of the Dead*. Secaucus, NJ: University Books. (Original work published 1895.)

Budge, E. A. W. (1989). *The Rosetta Stone*. New York: Dover. (Original work published 1929.)

Butler, J. (1993). *Bodies that Matter: On the Discursive Limits of "Sex."* New York: Routledge.

Campbell, J. (1973). *Hero with a Thousand Faces*. Princeton, NJ: Princeton University Press.

Carroll, B. J. (1993). Neurobiological dimensions of depression and mania. In J. Angst (Ed.), *The Origins of Depression: Current Concepts and Approaches* (pp. 163–186). Berlin: Springer-Verlag.

Clymer, A. (2002, December 27). U.S. revises sex information and the fight goes on. *New York Times*, p. A17.

Cornell, D. (1992). *Philosophy of the Limit*. New York: Routledge.

Damasio, A. (1994). *Descartes' Error: Emotions, Reason, and the Human Brain*. New York: G. P. Putnam's.

Damasio, A. (1999). *The Feeling of what Happens: Body and Emotion in the Making of Consciousness*. New York: Harcourt Brace.

Dawkins, E. (1989). *The Selfish Gene*. Oxford, U.K.: Oxford University Press.

Dennett, D. C. (1991). *Consciousness Explained*. Boston: Little, Brown.

Dickinson, E. (1924). *The Complete Poems*. Boston: Little, Brown.

Dostoyevsky, F. (1958). *The Double*. Bloomington: Indiana University Press. (Original work published 1846.)

Eccles, J. C. (1991). *Evolution of the Brain, Creation of the Self*. New York: Routledge.

Edelman, G. M. (1988). *Topobiology: An Introduction to Molecular Embryology.* New York: Basic Books.

Edelman, G. M. (1989). *The Remembered Present: A Biological Theory of Consciousness.* New York: Basic Books.

Edelman, G. M. (1992). *Bright Air, Brilliant Fire: On the Matter of the Mind.* New York: Basic Books.

Edelman, G. M. & Tononi, G. (2000). *A Universe of Consciousness: How Matter Becomes Imagination.* New York: Basic Books.

Edelman, G. M. (2004). *Wider than the Sky: The Phenomenal Gift of Consciousness.* New Haven, CT: Yale University Press.

Elsasser, W. M. (1998). *Reflections on a Theory of Organism: Holism in Biology.* Baltimore: Johns Hopkins University Press.

Foucault, M. (1980). *Power/Knowledge.* (G. Gordon, Ed.). New York: Pantheon.

Freud, S. (1994). *The Interpretation of Dreams.* (A. Brill, Trans.). New York: Barnes & Noble. (Original work published 1900.)

Gelernter, D. (1994). *The Muse in the Machine: Computerizing the Poetry of Human Thought.* New York: Free Press.

Glanz, J. (1997). Mastering the nonlinear brain. *Science, 277,* 1758–1959.

Goldstein, R. Z., & Volkow, N. D. (2002, October). Drug addiction and its underlying neurological basis: Neuroimaging evidence for the involvement of the frontal cortex. *American Journal of Psychiatry, 159*(10), 1642–1643.

Hameroff, S. H. (1998). Quantum computation in brain micro tubules? The Penrose–Hameroff "Orch-OR" model of consciousness. *Philosophical Transactions of the Royal Society of London A, 186,* 1869–1896.

Haraway, D. (1991). *Simians, Cyborgs, Women: The Reinvention of Nature.* London: Free Press.

Haykin, S. (1994). *Neural Networks: A Comprehensive Foundation.* New York: Macmillan.

Hebb, D. O. (1949). *The Organization of Behavior.* New York: Wiley.

Heidegger, M. (1977). *The Question Concerning Technology and other Essays.* (W. Lovitt, Trans.). New York: Harper & Row.

Irigaray, L. (1980). This sex which is not one. In E. Marks & I. de Courtrivon (Eds.), *New French Feminism: An Anthology* (pp. 99–106). Amherst, MA: University of Massachusetts Press.

James, W. (1890). *The Principles of Psychology.* New York: Dover.

Jung, C. G. (1958). *The Undiscovered Self.* New York: Penguin.

Kant, I. (1996). *Critique of Pure Reason.* Indianapolis, IN: Hackett. (Original work published 1781.)

Kaszniak, A. W. (1999). Consciousness. In D. Levenson, J. J. Ponzetti, & P. F. Jorgenson (Eds.), *Encyclopedia of Human Emotions.* New York: Macmillan.

Kramer, P. S. (1997). *Listening to Prozac: A Psychiatrist Explores Antidepressant Drugs and the Remaking of the Self.* New York: Penguin. (Original work published 1993.)

Kristeva, J. (1982). *Powers of Horror: An Essay on Abjection.* New York: Columbia University Press.

Lacan, J. (1982). *Ecrits: A Selection.* (A. Sheridan, Trans.). New York: Norton. (Original work published 1982.)

Mansfield, N. (2000). *Subjectivity: Theories of the Self from Freud to Haraway.* New York: New York University Press.

Marazziti, D. (2002). *La natura dell'amore.* Rome: Rizzoli.

Penrose, R. (1994). *Shadows of the Mind: A Search for the Missing Science of Consciousness.* New York: Oxford University Press.

Pratchett, T. (2001). *Thief of Time.* New York: Harper Collins.

Reiser, M. (2001). The dream in contemporary psychiatry. *American Journal of Psychiatry, 158*(3), 351–359.

Sanguineti, V. (1999). *Landscapes of My Mind*. Madison, CT: International Universities Press.

Scott, A. (1995). *Stairway to the Mind: The Controversial New Science of Consciousness*. New York: Springer-Verlag.

Scott, A. (2002). *Neuroscience: A Mathematical Primer*. New York: Springer-Verlag.

Searle, J. R. (1992). *The Rediscovery of the Mind*. New York: Cambridge University Press.

Shelley, M. (1998). *Frankenstein or the Modern Prometheus*. New York: Oxford World's Classics (Oxford University Press).

Sherrington, C. S. (1951). *Man on his Nature*. New York: Cambridge University Press. (Original work published 1940.)

Snell, B. (1982). *The Discovery of the Mind in Greek Philosophy and Literature*. New York: Dover.

Stevenson, R. (1998). *The Strange Case of Dr. Jekyll and Mr. Hyde*. New York: Oxford World's Classics (Oxford University Press).

Stolorow, R., Brandchaft, B., & Atwood, F. (1987). *Psychoanalytic Treatment: An Intersubjective Approach*. Hillsdale, NJ: Analytic Press.

Sullivan, H. S. (1953). *The Interpersonal Theory of Psychiatry*. New York: Norton.

Sutherland, S. S. (1989). *The International Dictionary of Psychology*. New York: Continuum.

Union of Concerned Scientists. (2004). *Scientific Integrity in Policymaking: An Investigation into the Bush Administration's Misuse of Science*. Cambridge, MA. www.ucsusa.org.

Valenstein, E. S. (1998). *Blaming the Brain: The Truth about Drugs and Mental Health*. New York: Free Press.

Wallace, B. A. (2000). *The Taboo of Subjectivity: Toward a New Science of Consciousness*. New York: Oxford University Press.

Wilshire, B. W. (Ed.) (1984). *William James: The Essential Writings*. Albany, NY: State University of New York.

Name Index

Subject Index

DISCARDED

CONCORDIA UNIVERSITY LIBRARIES
GEORGES P. VANIER LIBRARY LOYOLA CAMPUS